The Specialist Registrar Handbook

Second edition

D0299865

John Gatrell
BA(Hons) FIPD MIMgt
Deputy Head, The Business School, Bournemouth University

and

Tony White
PhD FRCS MB BS AKC
Consultant Otolaryngologist and Visiting Professor, Bournemouth University

Radcliffe Medical Press

© 2001 John Gatrell and Tony White

Reprinted 2004

Radcliffe Medical Press
18 Marcham Road, Abingdon, Oxon OX14 1AA

First edition 1999

British Library Cataloguing in Publication Data

A catalogue record for this book is available from the British Library.

ISBN 1 85775 464 6

Typeset by Joshua Associates Ltd, Oxford
Printed and bound by TJ International Ltd, Padstow, Cornwall

Contents

Foreword

There is a famous household reference book from Victorian times called *Enquire Within* where information can be found on all matters of a practical nature. The introduction went thus: 'Whether you wish to model a flower in wax; to study the rules of etiquette; to serve relish for breakfast or supper; to plan a dinner for a large party or a small one; to cure a headache; to make a will; to get married; to bury a relative; whatever you may wish to do, make, or to enjoy, provided your desire has relation to the necessities of domestic life, I hope you will not fail to *Enquire Within.*'

In many ways *The Specialist Registrar Handbook* fulfils a similar function for those preparing for career-grade posts in the present day National Health Service. It offers information that is outside the narrow confines of clinical knowledge and skill, and covers a broad range of important topics that are seldom taught in any formal sense. It explains what managers mean by such terms as quality, clinical governance and risk management. It explains how the NHS is funded and who makes decisions about such things. And it provides a framework for critical self-appraisal in terms of how to deal with all the people who might be encountered in the complicated environment of the largest civilian employer in Europe.

It is a shame that the title confines the readership to the specialist registrar grade, because the contents would educate and inform many other professional staff in the NHS, not least consultants. It is easy to imagine a trainee embarrassing a trainer with superior knowledge of NHS administration after reading this book. John Gatrell and Tony White are to be congratulated in recognising a gap and filling it in such a readable and informative way. This new and updated edition builds on the success of the first and undoubtedly heralds more to come.

John Lilleyman
President
Royal College of Pathologists
January 2001

Preface

We have met many doctors who expressed the wish that they had received training early in their careers in a wider range of non-clinical aspects of their work. Others, who are committed to continuing professional development, seek learning material that will help them to handle the wider issues that they confront on a day-to-day basis, and for which initial medical education failed to prepare them. Nick Black, Professor of Health Services Research in the London School of Hygiene and Tropical Medicine, when reviewing a book for the *BMJ* in 1998, wrote: 'Doctors have traditionally received little or no help in learning some of the most useful and important skills that they need, such as dealing with bereavement, organising their work, management and team skills . . .'.

The Specialist Registrar Handbook was written to address these and other needs revealed by our research. Since its publication we have been delighted with the positive feedback received from specialist registrars and other grades of doctors. Before the book was first published it was piloted extensively, using a wide range of doctors. Many comments were received which helped us to develop the final version. The following quotation is taken from a letter written to us by a specialist registrar. It reflects many of the responses we received and helps to explain the book's purpose.

> I found the book easy to read and, as a 'brand new' specialist registrar, interesting and relevant, since I have never received any training in these areas as an SHO. I think it is important that specialist registrars receive training in non-clinical and management-orientated skills rather than just the traditional exam-orientated clinical teaching.

Since the first edition, public perception of the external accountability of doctors has led the General Medical Council to introduce a system of revalidation. The impact of clinical governance has become clearer, and government initiatives have further affected the context in which doctors perform their work. These factors have been taken into account in this edition, which deals in more depth with quality and appraisal. Sections relating to the NHS context have been updated and medical negligence is also given more attention.

We hope you will find the book helpful as a means of supporting your continuing professional development.

John Gatrell
Tony White
January 2001

Acknowledgements

We remain especially grateful to Dr Hugh Platt, whose vision initiated and inspired this work.

We owe a debt to our colleagues in the Business School at Bournemouth University, particularly to Pam Corsie for providing high-quality support throughout various stages of the continuing development of the handbook. Our thanks are also due to those readers who took the trouble to contact us with suggestions for this second edition.

We wish to thank those who provided wisdom and guidance from various medical Royal Colleges, Postgraduate Deaneries, the Medical Defence Union, the NHSE, and hospital and primary care trusts. We freely acknowledge that some ideas may have been seeds sown during discussions with these people. We apologise if any reference is not attributed or is incorrectly acknowledged; any such errors are ours alone.

Particular thanks are due to Dr George Cowan and Dr Shelley Heard, North Thames Postgraduate Deanery, for their advice on appraisal and selection; Dr Clair du Boulay, Southampton University Hospital, for her guidance on revalidation; and Edward White, Southampton University School of Medicine, who wrote from his experience of undertaking research.

Not least, we are grateful to our wives, Susie and Anne, without whose support, tolerance and encouragement the whole project would not have been possible.

Introduction

This book has three main aims:

- to support the development of a range of skills related to effective professional performance
- to provide a basis for maximising learning opportunities throughout hospital-based training
- to serve as a source of useful information to specialist registrars and other doctors.

It is not always possible to rely on a colleague to give you support and instruction at the time you need it. Occasionally, it is difficult to ask – we are supposed to acquire knowledge of some aspects of our work through a kind of osmosis, but unfortunately this process cannot be relied upon. This handbook tries to provide the answers you think you ought to know, but do not like to ask for! It also seeks to help you develop new skills and capabilities that we know are relevant to professional careers. You may wish to dip into it to help you with a particular problem, or work through sections in order to learn more about particular aspects of your work.

Some kinds of learning can be achieved through reading textbooks, some through one-to-one instruction, and others are better undertaken in group training sessions. All require opportunity, an element of underpinning knowledge and a commitment to learn. This handbook is designed to fit in with your work and be relevant to everyday needs. It supplements other training, such as short courses, which may become available from time to time.

The contents of this book have not been imposed by any committee or individual, but have emerged from an extensive survey of doctors at all stages in their careers. The findings indicated that a wide range of non-clinical skills and knowledge was required if they were to be capable of working effectively. Recognition that the work of doctors encompasses much more than clinical activity is evident in the creation and continuing growth of the British Association of Medical Managers (BAMM), a membership organisation for doctors.

Other evidence exists in current training arrangements for doctors. Higher Trainee Assessment Forms from some of the Royal Colleges include the following characteristics:

- teaching competence, lecturing style, presentation skills and ability to answer questions
- ability to anticipate problems, lead others, team-build and motivate
- ability at routine administration
- grasp of hospital management and politics
- relationships with colleagues and ability to diffuse problems in the team, inspire confidence and establish rapport.

These characteristics are covered, with others, in the handbook. We hope you enjoy the experience of using this book and find it valuable.

Needs and experience change, and it would be helpful for your successors if you let us know things that need to be included, things that could be omitted, and things that need changing or moving from one part or section to another. This process of continuous development and review will ensure that it stays relevant to the needs of all doctors in future.

Learning objectives

Key learning objectives of the handbook are listed below. In order to derive maximum benefit from this book, you might find it helpful to start by familiarising yourself with its contents as a whole. If you believe you are already sufficiently competent in a particular area, study the Action points in the section. This will help you to decide if you need to do more in the area. You may feel that certain sections are irrelevant to you at this stage in your training. Put them to one side, but make a mental note to return to them later. The handbook will also act as a reference document into which you may dip as a need arises.

On completion of this handbook you should be better able to:

- identify your preferred learning style and make better use of learning opportunities
- organise your time in a way that enables you to cope with work and enjoy available leisure time
- delegate tasks to others in a way that helps to develop them and permits you to make better use of your own capabilities
- make effective presentations to small and large groups
- work effectively in a team

- lead others in the achievement of team goals
- understand and deal with conflict
- deal with stress in yourself and others
- contribute usefully and effectively to meetings
- instruct and train others in skills and knowledge aspects of clinical tasks
- appraise others in the context of training and revalidation
- present clear and concise formal reports and other written communications
- undertake research and prepare articles for publication
- present yourself to positive effect in the selection process
- understand the role of information technology in NHS administration
- deal with patients and close family members in breaking bad news and related matters
- request a post mortem
- appear at a coroner's inquest
- support, advise and help to develop colleagues
- identify the key aspects of quality service delivery
- understand the concept of clinical governance
- differentiate between audit and research and understand the application of audit to a range of settings
- reflect on your personal values in the context of your career and work as a doctor
- understand something of the current structure and history of the NHS.

Exploring your approach to working and learning

The aim of this chapter is to enable you to reflect on your approach to your work, to explore your preferred learning style and to assist you to manage your time effectively.

What type of doctor are you?

You may find it interesting to carry out a quick self-diagnostic questionnaire and assess your own values in the context of your work as a doctor. It will also be interesting for you to repeat it, shortly before or after you are appointed as a consultant, and reflect on the changes that have occurred.

This questionnaire is derived from Mascie-Taylor, Pedler and Winkless (1996), page 9 and is used with permission.

Read each statement and place a tick in the box corresponding to one option of the four presented that most applies to you.

Question	A	B	C	D
In the development of my work people would describe me as . . .				
. . . striving on behalf of the whole.			☐	
. . . uninvolved.	☐			
. . . a good corporate citizen.		☐		
. . . a fighter for my own service.				☐

Question	A	B	C	D
When I am a consultant I . . .				
. . . should not be seen to have to lead very often.	☐			
. . . should lead from the front (and not expect to be questioned a great deal).		☐		
. . . lead by creating a vision for the hospital and enthusing others.			☐	
. . . have an important role within my team.				☐
My colleagues would tend to say of me that . . .				
. . . I am the sort of person who is likely to initiate and deal with change.			☐	
. . . I can be relied upon to look after my patients and play my part in the team.				☐
. . . I am perhaps a bit of a character and occasionally selfish and pushy.		☐		
. . . they tend not to talk or know much about me.	☐			
As a consultant it will be important for me to . . .				
. . . look after my patients and be supportive of the hospital.				☐
. . . look after my patients and develop my service and specialty.		☐		
. . . look after my patients and avoid wasting time doing other things.	☐			
. . . look after my patients and contribute ideas for the development of the hospital.			☐	
I believe it is important for research to be carried out in the hospital . . .				
. . . so long as it does not interfere with patient care or divert one away from outside interests.	☐			
. . . so that doctors can treat patients more effectively.				☐
. . . so as to improve patient services the hospital offers and enhance its reputation.			☐	
. . . so that the reputation of individual doctors and their specialty is enhanced.		☐		
As a future consultant I . . .				
. . . should be a leader of my team where appropriate.				☐
. . . should be unconcerned to any great extent with leading others.	☐			
. . . should become a leader of my specialty.		☐		
. . . should be a leader in the hospital.			☐	
In my non-clinical working relationships with others in the hospital I . . .				
. . . single mindedly pursue the self-interest of my specialty.		☐		
. . . do not have many relationships with others.	☐			
. . . attempt to work with others to the best of my ability.				☐
. . . attempt to show others there is a brighter future.			☐	
In dealing with patients I . . .				
. . . resist any restriction that a shortage of resources might bring about.		☐		
. . . just get on with dealing with the individual.	☐			
. . . make sure the hospital as a whole responds, as well as possible, to the needs of patients.			☐	
. . . recognise there are issues beyond the individual patient.				☐

Question	A	B	C	D
When I attend a management course my interest would be in . . .				
. . . how to make a team work more effectively, contributing to others and the hospital.				☐
. . . leadership and strategic management.			☐	
. . . understanding the system so that I can get what I want.		☐		
. . . very little of what was on offer.	☐			
I believe the curriculum for medical students should comprehensively cover . . .				
. . . more medical topics and less of the 'social sciences'.		☐		
. . . methods of effective team working.				☐
. . . strategic management of the NHS.			☐	
. . . managing the doctor/patient relationship.	☐			
In terms of my leadership style I . . .				
. . . like to join with people and participate.				☐
. . . tell people what they need to know.		☐		
. . . consult, then seek to influence.			☐	
. . . have never really thought about it much.	☐			
Modern management practices in the NHS . . .				
. . . must be resisted at all times by the profession.		☐		
. . . have a useful place.				☐
. . . are only vaguely understood by me.	☐			
. . . offer the key to the future.			☐	
My view of managers in the NHS is that they . . .				
. . . are partners in the management of a complex organisation.			☐	
. . . are irrelevant to my practice.	☐			
. . . are an unnecessary imposition.		☐		
. . . have a part to play and contribution to make.				☐
In my view, purchasers . . .				
. . . should find the funds to enable my specialty to expand.		☐		
. . . should be seen as partners in the strategic development of our hospital.			☐	
. . . should ensure balance in developments even if it hits my specialty negatively.				☐
. . . seem very remote and beyond my sphere of influence.	☐			
As a consultant, financial considerations should . . .				
. . . be none of my concern.	☐			
. . . be of importance.		☐		
. . . be vigorously resisted if they get in the way of my service.	☐			
. . . have a part to play.				☐

Question	A	B	C	D

As a consultant, if I was invited by the Chief Executive to a meeting to discuss significant cost reductions which might affect my clinical practice, I would . . .

. . . either not attend the meeting or attend and say nothing. □ (C)

. . . attend, recognising that to resolve the issue requires a team-working approach. □ (D)

. . . attend in order to make positive suggestions for taking the hospital forward. □ (C)

. . . attend in order to minimise the effect on my specialty. □ (C)

In discussions about the resource implications of practice with my colleagues, I . . .

. . . accept that resource limitations are part of the ethical debate. □ (D)

. . . take the view that practice guidelines should not be influenced by resource implications. □ (B)

. . . persuade other clinicians of the need to seek solutions to such dilemmas. □ (C)

. . . tend not to venture a view. □ (A)

As a future consultant I would like my professional work to be recognised for . . .

. . . strongly influencing the direction of the hospital. □ (C)

. . . providing a good service. □ (D)

. . . solely my clinical work. □ (B)

. . . being influential in the profession. □ (C)

I feel that the purchaser/provider split . . .

. . . shifted power from doctors in a most inappropriate way. □ (C)

. . . emphasised the need for consultants in directorates to work together. □ (D)

. . . was irrelevant to my practice. □ (B)

. . . created hospitals that require strategic leadership. □ (C)

If it were suggested that the hospital in which I was working should merge with another in the interests of patient care, I would . . .

. . . only support the merger if I thought my own specialty would benefit. □ (C)

. . . contact my opposite numbers in the other unit to help forge an effective new alliance. □ (C)

. . . support the merger in the light of the common good. □ (D)

. . . recognise that I would have little influence over the outcome. □ (B)

My view of attending conferences is that they . . .

. . . can be useful for networking effectively with other influential doctors and managers. □ (C)

. . . are essential to meet and influence other important doctors in my specialty. □ (B)

. . . are not normally part of my life or practice. □ (A)

. . . are something I do in order to keep up-to-date. □ (D)

Question	A	B	C	D

The leadership of clinical services . . .
. . . rests with the doctor in so far as my patients are concerned.   ☐ (A)
. . . is a medical role with some important managerial implications.   ☐ (B)
. . . should be shared on the basis of professional expertise.   ☐ (D)
. . . is the doctor's right.   ☐ (C)

A primary care-led NHS . . .
. . . will make me work with other colleagues to meet GPs' needs.   ☐ (D)
. . . is doomed to failure since it removes power from those who really understand.   ☐ (B)
. . . is a piece of jargon which I don't really understand.   ☐ (A)
. . . represents a strategic opportunity for the hospital which should be embraced.   ☐ (C)

Consultant job plans are . . .
. . . helpful for consultants to work together.   ☐ (D)
. . . an unnecessary imposition by the management on consultant practice.   ☐ (B)
. . . unnecessary given the straightforward nature of consultant work.   ☐ (A)
. . . a useful tool in ensuring that objectives of a hospital are met.   ☐ (C)

What I admire most in my colleagues is . . .
. . . their ability to lead.   ☐ (D)
. . . the way they are not distracted from their daily clinical work.   ☐ (A)
. . . their ambition for themselves and their specialty.   ☐ (B)
. . . their being prepared to contribute to the team effort.   ☐ (C)

I would like to think that my obituary in the *BMJ* will say . . .
. . . I was first and last an outstanding clinician.   ☐ (A)
. . . I was primarily an outstanding medical manager.   ☐ (C)
. . . I was primarily outstanding in my specialty.   ☐ (B)
. . . I was primarily outstanding in working in a team for the good of the patient.   ☐ (D)

Analysis of your questionnaire

The ticks for your answers fall under columns headed A, B, C or D. Add up the total scores for the whole questionnaire for each column and enter into the following boxes:

A   B   C   D
☐   ☐   ☐   ☐

Your highest score suggests one of four possible positions doctors take with regard to the resolution of common dilemmas which arise in fulfilling their role. Doctors manage (at various levels) their personal practice in teams and groups, departments and units etc. Full details of the use of a Repertory Grid approach to this analysis can be found in Mascie-Taylor, Pedler and Winkless (1993), who produced four ideal-type descriptions or 'identikits'.

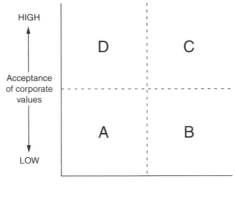

Figure 1.1 Types in relation to resources and corporate values.

The caricatures emerge with clarity but Type A turns out to include a variety of subtypes. A cautionary note. People vary in the way they respond to questionnaires by tending to score either low or high marks or go for the middle option. Also, each question is given equal weight so the salient questions for you may not be fairly represented. You need to remember these points, particularly if you are making comparisons with other people.

What type are you?

TYPE D – the TEAM PLAYER – 'the good corporate citizen'

Focus:

- primarily to the team but with awareness and interest in the whole organisation
- team leader, advising rather than leading the organisation.

Abilities and skills:

- takes leadership at team level and is prepared to accept it at corporate level
- plays by rules within corporate goals – building block of the organisation
- participative, co-operative, loyal, supportive, shares responsibilities and a team worker
- good interpersonal skills – good communicator
- economical with resources

- personable and well respected.

Beliefs and values:

- service orientation
- recognises added value and complementary skills of management
- democratic process, participation and consultation
- loyalty to medicine and medical values together with valuing the whole organisation.

The downside:

- the backbone of the organisation
- dedicated clinicians – the 'sort you'd like to take your mother to see'
- interested in playing their part in the whole
- lack confidence or have insufficient skills to be Type Cs
- less inclined to take risks than Type Cs
- prefer to avoid tough decisions
- may choose the quiet life
- may pursue outside interests
- may focus on the medical role
- less likely than Type Cs to take on formal management roles
- careful with resources
- may be self-sacrificing in meeting demands of others.

TYPE C – the LEADER – 'who strives on behalf of the whole'

Focus:

- commitment to the organisation
- wide view, broad vision and strategic thinking.

Abilities and skills:

- change agent – politically astute
- high interpersonal skills, influential, good communicator, good listener, assertive and can be tough
- manages resources on behalf of the whole
- develops people and teams
- manages conflict; constructive and supportive; tolerant of ambiguity and dilemmas.

Beliefs and values:

- quality, service and value for money requires doctors and managers to work together
- capability in the whole system is what counts

- pluralistic; different sources of loyalty are legitimate; conflict is inevitable, endemic and needs to be managed
- people (including self) are developing beings and can learn.

The downside:

- managers may regard you as too good to be true and lacking a 'shadow side'
- although Type Cs are often highly committed and very able leaders, Type Bs and perhaps Type As may see them as having 'gone over to the other side' or failed to make it in medicine and now seeking an alternative career
- some Type Cs may be Type Bs in temporary disguise, playing the corporate game in order to secure advantage. Others may indeed be more interested in personal career advancement than with rather altruistic 'good of the whole'. A strong motivation may be the desire to learn and explore new possibilities, not just of career but of person
- Type Cs are widely liked and respected for their leadership qualities, especially by Type Ds.

TYPE B – the INDEPENDENT – 'who fights for own patch'

Focus:

- me and my specialty
- me and my profession.

Abilities and skills:

- confident, dominant, determined – may be aggressive
- political skills, well connected and knows the 'right people'
- entrepreneurial, energetic and hard working
- uses conflict
- good ideas which are sometimes functional and sometimes dysfunctional for the organisation.

Beliefs and values:

- self-belief and self-worth
- individuality and individual excellence is what counts
- specialty is all important
- doctors don't need managing but do need administration
- rules are to be broken – or 'my rules'.

Downside:

- little in the way of corporate loyalty or values
- disinterested in corporate management
- see managers (at best) as a means of acquiring resources for their patch
- often lack sensitivity to others and may appear aloof, overbearing or arrogant

- arouse strong feelings of admiration, fear or dislike
- express themselves well in advancing their own work or specialty but poor at teamwork, chairing meetings or achieving agreement
- can be extrovert, convivial and amusing
- ability to command resources in the hospital or via external funding or university etc., while lacking an awareness and concern for the whole, often makes them the most difficult people to manage.

TYPE A – the CONTRACT CLINICIAN – 'uninvolved'

Focus:

- one-to-one patient care and clinical management with no interest, awareness or involvement beyond this.

This is probably a collection of subtypes. Classified as low on both corporate values and command of resources, this type has few abilities, skills, beliefs or values which are relevant from a managerial perspective.

The four subtypes are:

A1 The new starter
The very junior doctor on the way to Types B, C or D. May be naive, idealistic and dedicated with little awareness of how the hospital or health services work, and with little energy or attention to spare for learning the role.

A2 The disengager
Winding down and preparing to separate from the organisation through retirement, tiredness or ill health, etc.

A3 The contract worker
Personal doctor working 'nine to five' who doesn't want to get involved in anything outside one-to-one patient care. May have domestic responsibilities or consuming interests outside work. Does a job for the hospital within the strict limits of the contract.

A4 The isolate
The loner who may be good, bad or indifferent but is essentially unrecognised in terms of contribution. May work in a remote location or specialty, or be isolated for some other reason.

The downside:

- Type As have least impact because they contribute little to the organisation as a whole beyond their immediate task. This is not a commentary on them as people or as doctors – they may be effective or ineffective at that task. They may be learners or about to retire, have a limited contractual relationship with the organisation or a deep moral involvement in patient healthcare. They share a certain isolation from the run of events and may be candidates for further personal and professional development.

Action

Note your type now and reflect on what this means for you, your colleagues, the hospital and your future in healthcare. You may find it instructive to repeat this questionnaire in your last year as a specialist registrar (SpR) and consider how you have changed and why.

Learning and problem solving – what is your preferred learning style?

The Calman reforms, which introduced the concept of the SpR, are based on the idea that with more structured training using more appropriate methods, training could be not only shorter but better. This section seeks to give insight into some concepts behind teaching and learning. An understanding of the thinking behind training methods being used today, including those introduced by the surgical Royal Colleges, will help you to get the most from your learning opportunities. We think it would be helpful to introduce you to the work of Kolb, Rubin and McIntyre (1984).

Career development and the maintenance of professional competence demand that doctors maintain learning habits throughout their working lives. Most of us associate learning with the process we followed at school and university, when tutors, often through lectures to large groups of students, provided us with knowledge and concepts which we dutifully wrote down and memorised, and fed back in essays, project work and examination questions completed as a means of assessing our learning. End of term, end of year and final examinations helped to confirm the view that demonstrating learning involved satisfying others – our assessors – that we had grasped the necessary *concepts*.

Necessary for what though? 'Real life', as you will have probably already realised, in the form of daily work with patients, requires a different approach, where problem solving requires us to gain *experience*, quite different from the unreal world of classroom learning. The concept of learning as we came to know it during school and university often seems irrelevant now.

The concept of problem solving also suggests an active rather than passive process. In other words, the responsibility for problem solving rests with you, in contrast to teaching, in which the teacher is responsible (for the learning). The problem-solver must experiment, take risks and gain experience in order to address the problem.

This separation of *educational* learning and *work* learning sometimes leads to difficulties for doctors in the transition from medical school to work-based training. Our preferred approaches to learning are usually based on early, school-based experience, which does not always match later learning needs. In this section we will:

- illustrate this concept
- identify your preferred learning style
- show how various learning styles are relevant to different situations
- provide a model for learning which will help you to take full advantage of learning opportunities as they arise
- help you to understand why you find some kinds of learning more acceptable than others.

The following inventory describes how you learn – the way you find out about and deal with ideas and situations in your life. Different people learn best in different ways. The different ways of learning described in the survey are equally good. The aim is to describe how you learn, not to evaluate your learning ability. You might find it hard to choose the descriptions that best characterise your learning style. Keep in mind that there are no right or wrong answers – all the choices are equally acceptable.

Learning style inventory (LSI)

Source: Kolb, Osland and Rubin (1995) – used with permission (*see* Related reading, p. 23)

Instructions

There are nine sets of four descriptions listed in this inventory. Mark the words in each set that are most like you, second most like you, third most like you and least like you. Put a four (4) next to the description that is **most** like you, a three (3) next to the description that is **second** most like you, a two (2) next to the description that is **third** most like you and a one (1) next to the description that is **least** like you (4 = **most** like you; 1 = **least** like you). Be sure to assign a different rank number to each of the four words in each set. *Do not make ties.*

Example:

0   4___happy 3___fast 1___angry 2___careful

Some people find it easiest to decide first which word best describes them (4__happy) and then decide the word that is least like them (1__angry). Then you can give a (3) to that word in the remaining pair that is most like you (3__fast) and a (2) to the word that is left over (2__careful).

1	__discriminating	__tentative	__involved	__practical
2	__receptive	__relevant	__analytical	__impartial
3	__feeling	__watching	__thinking	__doing
4	__accepting	__risk taker	__evaluative	__aware
5	__intuitive	__productive	__logical	__questioning
6	__abstract	__observing	__concrete	__active
7	__present-oriented	__reflecting	__future-oriented	__pragmatic
8	__experience	__observation	__conceptualisation	__experimentation
9	__intense	__reserved	__rational	__responsible

Scoring instructions

The four columns of words correspond to the four learning style scales: **CE, RO, AC** and **AE**. To compute your scale scores, write your rank numbers in the boxes below only for the designated items. For example, in the third column (**AC**), you would fill in the rank numbers you have assigned to items 2, 3, 4, 5, 8 and 9. Compute your scale scores by adding the rank numbers for each set of boxes.

score items:	score items:	score items:	score items:
2 3 4 5 7 8	1 3 6 7 8 9	2 3 4 5 8 9	1 3 6 7 8 9
————————	————————	————————	————————
Total:	Total:	Total:	Total:
CE = ___	**RO** = ___	**AC** = ___	**AE** = ___

When the characteristics of learning and problem solving are combined, it is possible to come to a closer understanding of how people use their experience to develop concepts, rules and principles that guide their behaviour in new situations. The process can be conceived as a four-stage cycle as shown in Figure 1.2.

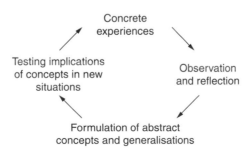

Figure 1.2 Four-stage cycle.

Concrete experience is followed by **observation and reflection** on the experience. These lead to the formation of **abstract concepts** and generalisations which are tested by **active experimentation** in the fourth stage. This leads to further experience and so on. The model shows learning as a continuously recurring cycle. All learning is relearning and all education is re-education. It may also be assumed that learning is shaped by personal needs and goals, which affect the ways in which we interpret experience. Thus, learning is likely to be erratic and inefficient when personal objectives are not clear.

Interpreting your scores on the learning style inventory

The LSI is a simple self-description test based on experiential learning theory. It is designed to measure your strengths and weaknesses as a learner in the four stages of the learning process. Effective learners use four different learning modes: concrete experience (**CE**), reflective observation (**RO**), abstract conceptualisation (**AC**) and active experimentation (**AE**).

One way to understand the meaning of your scores on the LSI is to compare them with the scores of others. Figure 1.3 gives the norms on the four basic scales (**CE**, **RO**, **AC** and **AE**) for 1933 (American) adults ranging from 18 to 60 years of age. About two-thirds of the group are men and the group as a whole is well educated (two-thirds have degrees or higher). A wide range of occupation and educational backgrounds are represented. They include teachers, engineers, managers, doctors and lawyers.

The raw scores for each of the four basic scales are marked on the crossed lines of the target. By marking your raw scores on the four scales and connecting them with straight lines, you can create a graphic representation of your learning style profile. The concentric circles on the target represent percentile scores for the normative group.

It should be emphasised that the LSI does not accurately define your learning style. It is an indication of how you see yourself as a learner. Your scores indicate which learning modes you emphasise in general. They may change from time to time and situation to situation.

The inventory is designed to give you some indication of which learning modes you tend to emphasise. No mode is better or worse than any other. Even a totally balanced profile is not necessarily the best. The key to effective learning is being competent in each mode when it is appropriate.

Orientation towards **concrete experience** suggests being involved in experiences and dealing with immediate human situations in a personal way. It emphasises *feeling* as opposed to *thinking*, and concern with the uniqueness and complexity of present reality as opposed to theories and models an intuitive, artistic approach as opposed to a systematic, scientific approach to problems. People with concrete

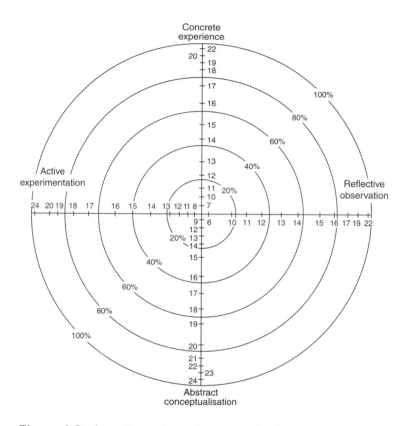

Figure 1.3   Learning style profile norms (© David A Kolb (1976)).

experience orientation enjoy (and are good at) relating to others. They can be good intuitive decision makers and function well in unstructured situations. They value highly relationships with people, being involved in real situations and keep an open-minded approach to life.

An orientation towards **reflective observation** emphasises understanding the meaning of ideas and situations by carefully observing and impartially describing them, as opposed to practical application. Such people enjoy thinking about the *meaning* of situations and ideas and are good at discovering their implications. They often look at things from different perspectives and appreciate different points of view. They value patience, impartiality and considered, thoughtful judgement and tend to rely on their own thoughts and feelings to form opinions.

Orientation towards **abstract conceptualisation** focuses on using logic, ideas and concepts. It emphasises thinking as opposed to feeling and is concerned with building general theories rather than intuitive understanding. Such people enjoy (and are good at) systematic planning, manipulation of abstract symbols and quantitative analysis. They value precision, the rigour and discipline of analysing ideas and the aesthetic quality of a neat conceptual system.

An orientation towards **active experimentation** focuses on actively influencing people and changing situations. It emphasises practical applications as opposed to reflective understanding, a pragmatic concern with what works as opposed to what is absolute truth. Such people enjoy (and are good at) getting things accomplished. They are willing to take some risk to achieve their objectives. They also value having an impact and influence on the environment around them and like to see results.

Action

Greater insight into your preferred learning style should provide you with a basis for exploiting learning opportunities. If possible, discuss your profile with that of colleagues. Compare and contrast them, and consider if it helps to explain your previous performance in learning situations and different subject areas.

Identifying your learning style type

It is useful to describe your learning style by a single data point that combines your scores on the four basic modes. This is accomplished by using the two combination scores: **AC** minus **CE** and **AE** minus **RO**. These scales indicate the degree to which you emphasise *abstract* over *concrete* and *action* over *reflection*, respectively.

The grid in Figure 1.4 has the raw scores for these two scales on the crossed lines (**AC** − **CE** on the vertical and **AE** − **RO** on the horizontal) and percentile scores based on the normative group on the sides. By marking your raw scores on the two lines and plotting their point of interception, you can find which of the four learning style quadrants you fall into. These four quadrants, labelled *accommodator*, *diverger*, *converger* and *assimilator*, represent the four dominant learning styles. If your **AC** − **CE** score was −4 and your **AE** − **RO** score +8, you would fall strongly in the accommodator quadrant. An **AC** − **CE** score of +4 and an **AE** − **RO** score of +3 would put you only slightly in the converger quadrant. The closer your data point is to the point where the lines cross, the more balanced your learning style. If your data point is close to any of the four corners, this indicates that you rely heavily on one particular learning style.

The following is a description of the characteristics of the four basic learning styles based both on research and clinical observation of these patterns of LSI scores.

The *convergent* learning style relies primarily on the dominant learning abilities of abstract conceptualisation and active experimentation. The greatest strength of this approach lies in problem solving, decision making and the practical application of ideas. This learning style is called the converger because a person with this style

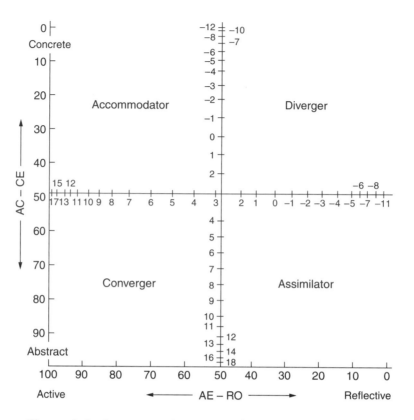

Figure 1.4 Learning style type grid (© David A Kolb (1976)).

seems to do best in such situations as conventional intelligence tests where there is a single correct answer or solution to a question or problem. In this learning style, knowledge is organised in such a way that, through hypothetical–deductive reasoning, it can be focused on specific problems. Liam Hudson's research on individuals with this style of learning shows that convergent persons are controlled in their expression of emotion. They prefer dealing with technical tasks and problems rather than with social and interpersonal issues. Convergers often specialise in the physical sciences. This learning style is characteristic of many engineers and technical specialists.

The *divergent* learning style has the opposite strengths of the convergent style, emphasising concrete experience and reflective observation. The greatest strength of this orientation lies in imaginative ability and awareness of meaning and values. The primary adaptive ability in this style is to view concrete situations from many perspectives and to organise many relationships into a meaningful 'Gestalt'. The emphasis in this orientation is on adaptation by observation rather than by action. This style is called diverger because a person of this type performs better in situations that call for generation of alternative ideas and implications, such as a 'brainstorming' idea session. Persons oriented toward divergence are interested in people and tend to be imaginative and feeling-oriented. Divergers have broad cultural interests and tend to specialise in the arts. This style is characteristic of individuals from humanities and liberal arts backgrounds. Counsellors, organisation development specialists and personnel managers tend to be characterised by this learning style.

In *assimilation,* the dominant learning abilities are abstract conceptualisation and reflective observation. The greatest strength of this orientation lies in inductive reasoning, in the ability to create theoretical models and in assimilating disparate observations into an integrated explanation. As in convergence, this orientation is less focused on people and more concerned with ideas and abstract concepts. Ideas, however, are judged less in this orientation by their practical value. Here it is more important that the theory be logically sound and precise. This learning style is more characteristic of individuals in the basic sciences and mathematics rather than the applied sciences. In organisations, persons with this learning style are found most often in the research and planning departments.

The *accommodative* learning style has the opposite strengths of assimilation, emphasising concrete experience and active experimentation. The greatest strength of this orientation lies in doing things, in carrying out plans and tasks, and in getting involved in new experiences. The adaptive emphasis of this orientation is on opportunity seeking, risk taking and action. This style is called accommodation because it is best suited for those situations in which one must adapt oneself to changing immediate circumstances. In situations where the theory or plans do not fit the facts, those with an accommodative style will most likely discard the plan or theory. With the opposite learning style (assimilation), one would be more likely to disregard or re-examine the facts. People with an accommodative orientation tend to solve problems in an intuitive trial and error manner, relying on other people for information rather than on their own analytic ability. Individuals with accommodative learning styles are at ease with people but are sometimes seen as impatient and pushy. This person's educational background is often in technical or practical fields, such as business. In organisations, people with this learning style are found in 'action-oriented' jobs, such as marketing or sales positions.

Making effective use of your time

Time is a remarkable commodity. No matter how we waste time today, tomorrow's entitlement remains untouched. Most junior doctors recognise the problem of time management. You need to organise your time and clinical work around structured sessions, clinics, ward rounds and theatre sessions. You need to organise yourself and your tasks when you are on call, as well as your time on call itself. Your work makes multiple demands on your time, such as writing up discharge summaries, dictating notes from your most recent clinic, preparing a paper to present to the firm at the weekly journal club and perhaps a promise to read through a paper for a colleague. Then there is your private life outside work and finding time for family and friends – even for yourself! Few have found a simple solution. Most do their best, but some are definitely better at this than others. How well do you use *your* time? Try to answer the following as honestly as you can.

Place a cross (×) under the appropriate heading for each item.

Item	Strongly agree	Slightly agree	Slightly disagree	Strongly disagree
1 My work tends to mount up.				
2 I tend to put off large or unpleasant jobs.				
3 I find it difficult to say 'No' to requests from others.				
4 I waste a lot of time in meetings.				
5 I have to start and stop jobs frequently.				
6 I spend too much time moving from place to place.				
7 I have too much paperwork to deal with.				
8 I spend a great deal of time on the telephone.				
9 I always seem to be trying to do too many things at the same time.				
10 I never have time to prioritise tasks – I deal with problems as they arise.				
11 The only way I can cope is by taking paperwork home with me.				
12 I seldom have time to just sit and think.				
13 Colleagues would describe me as disorganised.				
14 I tend to mislay papers.				
15 Other people always seem to come to me for advice.				
16 I generally feel out of control of my career and life.				

Action

List the items which you marked as strongly agree.

-
-
-
-
-
-

Now take each of these items and consider *why* this is the case. What do *you* do, and what do *others* do, to contribute to your problem? It may be helpful to discuss it with colleagues or friends. Try to identify the work-related and personal consequences of each 'strongly agree' item. Next, prioritise these items in the order in which you would like to resolve them. Take the first item and write down the action you need to take to deal with the problem. Specify the action and support you need from others in achieving this. Do this for each of the other items.

The following guidelines may help you in setting a framework for resolving problems which arise in your use of time.

Goal setting

As a doctor and SpR, you need to manage simultaneous tasks, such as dealing with an emergency admission while managing another patient about whom you are concerned and who is located on a different ward. This is before you take account of your private life. The first thing to recognise is that, when thinking about organising your life, it is unhelpful to separate work and non-work.

Take a sheet of paper and write down your 'foreseeable life goals'. These are likely to be attainable within the next two or three years. Think of them as starting from now. They might be personal, family, social, career, financial, community and spiritual. Work quickly, without limiting your ambitions.

Next, review and refine these goals into statements that imply action. Some may be immediate, e.g. 'spend more time with my family'. Defining and securing your career objectives are likely to figure large. Others may require considerable balancing of resources and long-term planning, such as investing to secure early retirement. Some may be unrealistic and so should be disregarded at this stage.

Prioritise your goals. This involves taking decisions about yourself. Take into account your own values and circumstances. It can be difficult, but not as difficult as living without purpose. They will all be important, but some will be more important than others. Use them to develop your approach to time management.

Develop a sense of time. How do you *really* spend your day?

Analyse your working day by keeping a time log for a few days. You can use an ordinary desk diary. Record the activity in which you are engaged at 15-minute intervals throughout the day. This can be frightenly revealing of the time spent on various activities of which you were not aware.

List the activities and record the time spent on each in a typical week. Ask yourself if this reflects your priorities. Are there activities that take up time but contribute little or nothing? What would happen if you stopped doing them completely? How much of your time do you keep to use at your discretion? Are you spending time on work that could be delegated to others?

Planning

Define your goals for personal development and professional accomplishment for the coming year. Write them in a way that will allow you to measure your success in achieving them. Effective planning is impossible without a diary system. There are many options, including electronic personal organisers, wall charts and desk diaries. Choose the one that suits you. Set aside time (between 10 and 30 minutes) at the beginning of each day to list your tasks and prioritise them. You may find it helpful to use a simple system of letters or stars to indicate priority, for example:

*** *must* be done today
** *should* be done today
* *might* be done today.

It is crucial to understand the difference between tasks that are *urgent* and those that are *important*. Urgent but unimportant tasks should be done quickly, but given a small amount of your time. Important, non-urgent tasks can be scheduled for later in the day, week or month and given sufficient space in your diary to complete them properly at the first sitting. Some tasks will be a mixture of both.

Work through your list, completing each task before moving on to the next. Set a time limit for each task based on its priority. As a registrar, clearly some of your time may be largely outside your control. But not all of it. You will be surprised to find how much you do control. Use your daily planning session to make best possible use of the time you are able to influence. Do not worry if, at the end of the day, you have not completed all your tasks. Simply delete those that are no longer necessary and transfer the rest to your list for the following day.

Working routines

Incoming paperwork should be handled only once. Don't put a pathology or X-ray report down until you have decided what action to take, even if only to ask for advice. Do not put a letter down until you have written or dictated a reply. If you really cannot act immediately, *do something*, even if it is just to decide *when* you will take action.

Writing clearly, simply and concisely is essential for effective, first-time communication. Consider the purpose of your communication, jot down key points then arrange them in a logical order. Use short sentences, avoiding jargon and formal language.

Reading is an important method of personal development for doctors. Develop the following habits when dealing with your paperwork. Scan lengthy documents before deciding whether you need to read them all. Perhaps look only at the introduction and summary or conclusions. Highlight key points so that you can refer back to them easily. 'Speed-reading' can be useful for those with many large documents to absorb, but is no substitute for good judgement in deciding what to read!

Telephones save time when used appropriately. Try recording your telephone use during one week. You may be surprised at the total time taken up. Before using the telephone, make a quick note of what you wish to say. Keep the conversation on track and bring it to a polite end when you have completed your business. Better still, delegate others to make, answer or return telephone calls for you. Mobile phones can be a mixed blessing. Ask yourself 'would (or does) having one give me more, or less, control over my life?'

Avoid procrastination. Set starting times for tasks you might be tempted to put off. Forget about finishing the task – concentrate on starting it. Make your deadlines public. Reward yourself for completing unpleasant tasks. Learn to say 'No' to unreasonable or low-priority requests from others. It takes practice to do this assertively, and without offending.

Working with others

Meetings can waste a lot of time. First, ask yourself if the meeting is necessary, or if you need to attend. If you have called the meeting, prepare an agenda, set a time limit and communicate these to others before it starts. Encourage them to prepare for the meeting. Discourage irrelevant discussion. There is a separate section on meetings in this handbook.

Delegation can be painful. Giving away tasks you enjoy, or feel you cannot trust to others, may be the only way to release time for what you need to do to achieve results. There is more on delegation in Chapter 2.

Saying 'No' to impossible or unnecessary tasks is often more difficult than it should be. We are brought up to acquiesce to our seniors, rather than challenge them, and this creates habits that are nearly impossible to break. Assertive behaviour is also dealt with in the next chapter.

Planning working rotas, partial and full shifts

Good continuity of care does not just happen, it has to be planned, implemented and managed if you are to make best use of your time. Here are some key points which might enable you to do this.

Ensure:

- there is protected time for the handover of staff, with an overlap of 15–30 minutes to allow for adequate communication
- information is relayed about all patients, not just the sick ones, placing you in a position to judge easily changes in patients' conditions
- you keep a written record of plans. This prevents you from forgetting something important due to the pressure of a new emergency. Provide yourself with a daily written update.

There are implications for all rotas operating within a specialty. For example, there is little point in the senior house officers (SHOs) handing over in exemplary fashion without the pre-registration house officers (PRHOs) or registrars being involved. Essentially, it is about good communication. You can improve your own work simply by taking a little time and trouble, for instance in paying attention to communication at handover.

Setting up this sort of organisation in a department, ensuring there is support, and bringing together the relevant medical and non-medical personnel is an exercise which will require consultant involvement. Consultants, in turn, will need the support and help of senior nurses and possibly managers. As a junior doctor, your most important role in improving work will be in selling the issue to your peers, particularly to your senior colleagues.

Action

Think back over the last fortnight.

- When starting on-call periods, have you always felt adequately briefed about the in-patients under your care?

- When coming on duty in the morning, when and how have you learned about new patients admitted over the on-call period?

- When going off duty in the evening, have you and your colleagues always fully briefed the on-call team about your patients?

Related reading

Buzan T (1989) *Use Your Head*. BBC Books, London.

Kolb DA, Osland JS and Rubin IM (1995) *Organizational Behaviour – an experiential approach* (6e). Prentice-Hall, Englewood Cliffs, New Jersey.

Mascie-Taylor HM, Pedler MJ and Winkless AJ (1993) *Doctors & Dilemmas: a study of 'ideal types' of doctor/managers and an evaluation of how these could support values of clarification for doctors in the health service*. NHSTD, Bristol.

Mascie-Taylor HM, Pedler MJ and Winkless AJ (1996) *Doctors & Dilemmas Workbook. A self-development programme of values clarification, dilemma resolution and effective action for doctors in the health service*. NHSTD, Bristol.

2

Managing the 'day-to-day'

The aim of this chapter is to develop your awareness of a range of aspects of dealing with people at work.

It provides underpinning knowledge for developing your skills in areas such as leadership and teamwork.

You cannot learn to lead and influence others just by reading a book – but it does help to have some background information. Much of this chapter is useful pre-reading for related training workshops.

Leading teams

Doctors usually work as part of a team, and this helps emphasise the importance of leadership. As your clinical responsibility grows, so does your need to lead and direct others. Leadership is about interpersonal skills and involves getting people to do things willingly.

Do you (have to) possess the right personality traits?

A traditional view of leadership held that a few people were born with special powers and aptitudes that made them natural leaders. These included enthusiasm, self-assurance, initiative, intelligence and so on. Studies of effective leaders have raised doubts about this view, research having failed to identify a consensus on such traits, particularly as many notably successful leaders are deficient in a significant proportion of the defined traits. While recognising the importance of personal qualities, attention is now directed to the behaviour and competence of leaders rather than inherent personal characteristics. Leadership is thus a complex process involving a range of skills which can be acquired through learning and practice.

Is leadership a matter of style?

Styles of leadership are usually defined as ranging between 'authoritarian' and 'democratic'. Five separate styles have been defined.

- Tells
  – the leader chooses the course of action to be followed, communicates it to subordinates and expects acceptance without debate.
- Sells
  – the leader anticipates the possibility of resistance from subordinates and attempts to persuade them of the merits of a decision.
- Consults
  – the leader presents a problem to the team and invites suggestions and advice before making a decision.
- Participates
  – the leader joins the group in arriving at a decision, inviting the group to assist in defining the problem.
- Delegates
  – sometimes referred to as 'empowerment', the leader develops staff and creates an environment of trust in which subordinates accept responsibility for problem solving and decision making.

The difference between one style and another often reflects the power relationship between the leader and the led. Authoritarian leaders have power and hold on to it, using it to direct and control the work behaviour of their subordinates. They retain the right to make decisions, to reward and punish. More democratic styles lead to delegation of decision making, or at least to sharing authority and control.

Some writers argue that people are more productive when working in a democratic environment. They reason that supportive styles of leadership help to create job satisfaction, reducing grievances and intergroup conflict. Some doubt, however, that such participative styles of leadership are always effective in enhancing group performance. Sometimes circumstances demand a directive style, for example in life or death situations. Style alone is insufficient as a determining factor, although it is important.

The following questionnaire should help you to identify your own style. When completing it, try to place yourself in a situation in which you might have to lead, even if this is not your normal role.

Task/process leadership questionnaire

Source: Pfeiffer and Jones (1974) – used with permission (*see* Related reading, p. 54).

The objective of this questionnaire is to identify your leadership style through your relative concern for tasks or people, and locate it in terms of three types of leadership: individual, group or shared.

Directions
The following items describe some aspects of leadership behaviour. Respond to each item according to how you would most likely act if you were the leader of a team or group. You could think of yourself in a group at work, or in a social, hobby or sports group with a task to carry out.

Circle whether you would most likely behave in the described way:

always **(A)**, frequently **(F)**, occasionally **(O)**, seldom **(S)** or never **(N)**.

	Item number	
I would most likely act as the spokesman of a group.	1	A F O S N
I would encourage team members to stay late to finish a task.	2	A F O S N
I would allow team members complete freedom in the way they worked.	3	A F O S N
I would encourage team members to use standard procedures.	4	A F O S N
I would allow team members to use their judgement in solving problems.	5	A F O S N
I would stress trying to be ahead of competing groups.	6	A F O S N
I would speak as representative of the group.	7	A F O S N
I would nag members for greater effort.	8	A F O S N
I would try out my ideas.	9	A F O S N
I would let people do their work the way they think best.	10	A F O S N
I would work hard to get praise.	11	A F O S N
I would tolerate delay and uncertainty.	12	A F O S N
I would speak for the group if there were outsiders present.	13	A F O S N
I would keep the work moving at a rapid pace.	14	A F O S N
I would let people loose on a job and allow them to get on with it.	15	A F O S N
I would settle any conflicts if they occurred.	16	A F O S N
I would get swamped with details.	17	A F O S N
I would represent the group at outside meetings.	18	A F O S N
I would be reluctant to allow the group any freedom of action.	19	A F O S N
I would decide what should be done and how it should be done.	20	A F O S N
I would push for maximum effort.	21	A F O S N
I would let some people have control which I could have kept.	22	A F O S N
Things usually turn out as I predict.	23	A F O S N
I would allow people a high degree of initiative.	24	A F O S N
I would assign people to particular tasks.	25	A F O S N

I would be happy to make changes.	26	A F O S N
I would ask people to work harder.	27	A F O S N
I would trust the group members to exercise their judgement.	28	A F O S N
I would arrange how the work was to be done.	29	A F O S N
I would not explain my reasons.	30	A F O S N
I would persuade the group of the advantages of my ideas.	31	A F O S N
I would allow the group to set their own pace.	32	A F O S N
I would urge my group to better their previous efforts.	33	A F O S N
I would not consult the group.	34	A F O S N
I would ask that people used only approved methods.	35	A F O S N

$$P = \underline{\hspace{1cm}} \qquad T = \underline{\hspace{1cm}}$$

Scoring the questionnaire is reasonably straightforward as long as you follow the instructions below step-by-step.

Scoring is as follows:

1 circle the item number for items 8, 12, 17, 18, 19, 30, 34 and 35
2 write the number 1 in front of a circled item number if you responded **S** (seldom) or **N** (never) to that item
3 also write a number 1 in front of item numbers not circled if you responded **A** (always) or **F** (frequently)
4 circle the number 1s you have written in front of the following items: 3, 5, 8, 10, 15, 18, 19, 22, 24, 26, 28, 30, 32, 34 and 35
5 count the circled number 1s. This is your score for *concern for people*. Record the score in the blank following the letter **P** at the end of the questionnaire
6 count the uncircled number 1s. This is your score for *concern for tasks*. Record this number in the blank following the letter **T**.

Now follow the instructions below to plot your **T–P** leadership style profile.

To determine your style of leadership, mark your score on the concern for task dimension (**T**) on the left-hand arrow in Figure 2.1. Next, move to the right-hand arrow and mark your score on the concern for people dimension (**P**). Draw a straight line that intersects the **P** and **T** scores. The point at which the line crosses the shared leadership arrow indicates your position on that dimension.

A high score on the **T** dimension and a low **P** score indicates a strong tendency to focus on getting the job done, perhaps at the expense of maintaining good working relations with the team. A high **P** and low **T** score probably means that team members are at ease with your style, although they might prefer more direction at times even at the expense of having an easy time. The higher your score on the middle (shared) dimension, the more you are likely to be able to adjust your style to suit situations where either a 'telling' style is more appropriate, or one in which you involve the team in decision making.

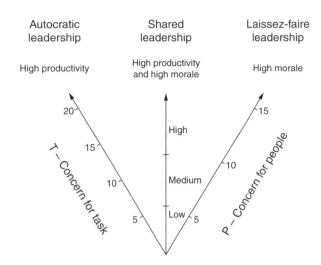

Figure 2.1   Shared leadership results from balancing concern for task and concern for people.

Good leaders adopt the right style, taking into account the situation!

Effective leaders get the task done while maintaining good working relationships with their colleagues. Appropriate leadership style is about finding the balance between task-oriented and relationship-oriented leadership behaviour.

* Task-oriented behaviour focuses on directing the actions of others, defining their roles and setting goals for them.
* Relationship-oriented behaviour concerns the extent to which the leader engages in listening, encouraging and supporting group members.

It is these two dimensions that produce the five leadership styles set out in Figure 2.2.

Choice of leadership style is not only dependent on the situation but also the maturity of the group. To review those styles again we can now say:

Telling is suited to immature groups which need high levels of guidance and structure to get the task done and are less in need of relationship building. It can also be the only way to lead in a crisis when the outcome might be life threatening. When leading a team dealing with a cardiac arrest, for example, there is little time or opportunity to debate alternative courses of action.

Selling emphasises both relationship and task behaviours and is suited to groups that have growing maturity and are in need of support through a team-building process, but need to be regularly reminded of the task. For example, if you decide

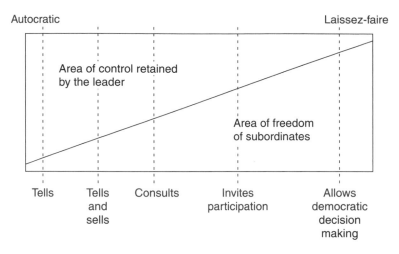

Figure 2.2 A continuum of leadership styles.

you would like to arrange a mess dinner or medical school year reunion and set out to persuade colleagues of the attractiveness of your idea.

Consulting allows the leader to maintain fairly close control while permitting the group to have an influence on practice and procedures. By listening to the suggestions of team members, the leader can often arrive at better decisions.

Participating emphasises two-way communication and support, but allows the team freedom to make decisions that influence outcomes. This can create a sense of achievement and commitment to the task, but generally depends on team members being well trained with a good understanding of team objectives. A decision to undertake a group or departmental audit project, for example, would require cooperation from all group members. Involving everyone in the decision would most likely achieve this.

Delegating can be used only with mature, well-trained teams capable of managing their own tasks and relationships. The leader's role is more 'hands off', while retaining accountability for results. This might include enlisting the help of SHOs, nurses or other colleagues to manage an influx of work for which you are responsible.

Transformational leadership

We all have a preferred style we tend to revert to when under pressure, but how can our leadership qualities and skills be developed? Assuming that the views outlined above are valid, it is *how you deal with people* rather than *what you are* that makes the difference. Current thinking on leadership emphasises the role of the leader as one who influences, generates change and develops confidence in followers to take on responsibility for their own work outcomes.

This approach has come to be known as transformational leadership. Such leaders appeal to higher motives in their followers and focus on positive values when discussing team objectives. They work from a vision of the future, rather than dependence on past history. This type of leader has been referred to as one who commits people to action, converts followers into leaders and converts leaders into agents of change.

There are three steps in leading organisational change. The first is recognition of the need for change. Effective leaders transmit this awareness to colleagues and followers and thus create a mood for change. The second stage is the communication of a new vision which encompasses the long- and short-term needs of the organisation. Avoiding quick-fix solutions is critical to success. Finally, the leader institutionalises the change by establishing new cultures and procedures, and by restructuring communication channels.

Getting results through others

Understanding what motivates people to achieve good results

Performance of anyone at work is dependent on three variables: their *ability*, which is a combination of aptitude and development; tools and facilities must be available, so they have the *opportunity*; and they must be *motivated*. In effect performance is the product of ability and motivation.

Good leaders understand what motivates people and act to get the best from them. They must also harness those energies towards the successful achievement of goals. Motivation (in this context) is concerned with why people choose a particular course of action and persist in that action in preference to others. The underlying concept of motivation is the existence of *needs* which give rise to *drive* and *action* in order to achieve desired *goals* – thus meeting these needs and creating *satisfaction*.

Human needs were said by Maslow in 1943 to be arranged in a hierarchy, with basic needs dominating higher order needs until the former are reduced. His model is often presented as in Figure 2.3.

Physiological needs include food, water and warmth – the basic requirements of survival. Safety and security needs are met through freedom from the threat of physical attack, protection from deprivation, and predictability and orderliness. Social needs are met by a sense of belonging, friendships and the giving and receiving of love. Esteem is focused on the self and involves the desire for confidence, status and the respect of others. Self-fulfilment (described by Maslow as self-actualisation) is the realisation of one's full potential. This may vary widely

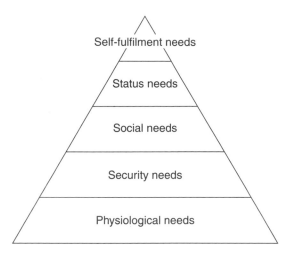

Figure 2.3   Maslow's hierarchy of needs.

from one individual to another. Some authors have suggested that a sixth need, which follows self-fulfilment, is self-awareness.

Maslow argues that these needs are hierarchical, and a need which is satisfied is no longer a motivator. Hence, as lower level needs are met, so the driving force of behaviour becomes the higher need. Needs do not have to be fully met. There is a gradual emergence of a higher level need as lower level needs become more satisfied. He also makes it clear that the hierarchy applies to most (not all) people. It is not necessarily a fixed order. Exceptions will be evident. Some people, driven by a creative and self-actualising urge, will ignore more basic needs. Others, with high ideals or values, may become martyrs and give up everything for the sake of their beliefs. It follows that, in order to provide motivation for changes in behaviour, a leader must direct attention to the next higher level of need.

Maslow's theory is difficult to test empirically. Attempts that have been made give only tentative support. The theory has been influential, nonetheless, perhaps because of its simplicity and universality.

The work of McClelland in 1976 led to a further content theory of motivation. He and his colleagues identified three main arousal-based, socially developed motive forces: affiliation, power and achievement. These correspond broadly to Maslow's highest order needs for love and security, esteem and self-actualisation. Their relative impact on behaviour varies with each individual. It was also possible to identify differences according to occupation. McClelland identified three common characteristics as a result of follow-up research focused on individuals with a high need for achievement. You may recognise them in some of your colleagues:

- a preference for personal responsibility
- the setting of achievable goals
- the desire for concrete feedback on performance.

These individuals like to be personally responsible for solving problems and getting results. They also like to attain success through their own efforts, rather than as a member of a team. The recognition of others is not as important as their own sense of accomplishment. A second characteristic is the tendency to set moderate achievement goals and take calculated risks. If the task is too difficult or risky, the chances of success would be reduced. If the task is too easy or safe, there would be little sense of achievement from success. Thirdly, feedback on performance should be prompt, clear and unambiguous. It helps to confirm success and give the sense of satisfaction that comes with achievement.

A second 'family' of motivational theories emphasises the study of process, rather than content. These seek to provide a better understanding of the relationship between variables that influence work behaviour. Process models are generally more able to accommodate individual differences. Among the best known is 'expectancy theory'. It emphasises an individual's perception of the probability that particular outcomes will result from specific courses of action. The model which is best known is based on three variables: valence, instrumentality and expectancy.

Valence is defined as the attractiveness of, or preference for, a particular outcome to an individual. If a person has a preference for a particular outcome, valence is positive. Where avoidance of a particular outcome is preferred, valence is negative. If the person is indifferent to the outcome, valence is zero. Valence is the expected satisfaction, and is distinguished from the value attached to the actual outcome, once achieved.

Instrumentality is best understood if we distinguish between first and second level outcomes. First level outcomes refer to actual performance in the work. For some, this will be an end to be valued for its own sake as 'a job well done'. For others, the valence of the performance outcomes is determined by the second level outcomes, which may for example, be derived from the financial gains resulting from satisfactory completion of the task. Second level outcomes are need related. Instrumentality is the extent to which first level outcomes lead to second level outcomes.

Expectancy is a perception of the probability that the choice of a particular action will lead to the desired outcome. It relates effort expended to the achievement of first level outcomes. This model, as with others derived from it, is useful in explaining the process by which people weigh and evaluate the attractiveness of different alternatives, before committing themselves to specific courses of action. The models do not, however, reflect the actual decision-making steps taken by an individual.

Studies of goal-oriented behaviour provide a further insight into motivation. Goal setting may be viewed as a motivational technique rather than a theory. A number of organisational systems emphasise the importance of agreeing work goals with employees, whose behaviour is thought to be determined by their goals. People's values give rise to emotions and desires which they strive to satisfy through their responses and actions. Goals direct work behaviour and performance and lead to certain consequences or feedback. People with specific, measurable goals will perform better than those without. Also, those with difficult but achievable goals will perform better than those whose goals may be easily achieved.

In general, theories and models of motivation are unable to provide universal solutions to the challenge of motivating people at work. They do, however, help us to understand the complexity of the process, taking us away from management approaches linked to fear and punishment, common among traditional managers earlier in the twentieth century.

Developing team spirit

There are many kinds of team, some permanent, such as committees, and some temporary, such as task forces and working groups. A good example of teamwork is the surgical team that includes the surgeon and anaesthetist together with their juniors, nurses, ODAs and others. Each is specialised and knows that each individual's success is dependent on the work of other team members. Bringing together the right number of people to work together does not necessarily make an effective team. This takes time.

Team building and developing team spirit

Initially, there may be confusion over members' roles and authority. Although there may be a nominal leader, others play leadership roles at times. Members gradually identify their roles but sometimes as individuals working together rather than as a team. Conflicts and interactions occur as personal ideas and agendas are sorted. Gradually the group comes to see itself no longer as a collection of individuals but as a group that has its own identity. There may even be experimentation with new roles. The group usually dies when the task has been completed and there may be feelings of sadness or even grief. If the task changes, some members leave and others join. So the cycle continues, and it is important to be aware of the dynamics of group behaviour.

There are said to be four stages in the development of a team. Obviously, it is seldom this simple if individuals leave and others join. This also disrupts the process of team building. Some teams may never develop into a mature team, for a variety of reasons which may be to do with the mix of personalities within the team or the transient nature of the work. There is no particular timing to the stages –

although they may be accelerated if attention is paid to helping the team through the four stages of growth.

- Forming
  – this is the early, testing stage, with members being polite, watchful and guarded. Members try to learn about each other and may begin to project their personality by giving formal information about themselves.
- Storming
  – there may be some confusion in the team (particularly about roles), with controlled conflict and confrontation and difficulties in agreeing tasks and goals, and with some team members opting out.
- Norming
  – the team starts to get organised and develop its skills, establishing roles and procedures, giving feedback and confronting issues that are perceived to affect performance.
- Performing
  – eventually the team may mature to be resourceful, flexible, effective and supportive.

The characteristics of a fully mature team are listed below.

- Team goals are clear and agreed.
- Information flows freely between members.
- Relationships between members are supportive, trusting and respectful.
- Conflict is regarded as natural and helpful, but concerns issues not people.
- The atmosphere is participative, open, non-threatening and non-competitive.
- Decisions are by consensus, although the team concedes authority to individual members to make decisions when it would be most helpful to do so.

Remember, it does not follow that if a group of people work together for sufficient time, a mature team will inevitably develop. Nor is there is a single approach to team building that is likely to work for all teams. One view is that the right mixture of personalities to make an effective team needs to be brought together in the first place. This, of course, is not usually possible, since hospital teams are usually decided by the availability of staff at the time the team is formed. Perhaps the most helpful thing to remember is that teams do not naturally fall into maturity – they need help, either from informed insiders or from someone who understands the mechanics of team building and can facilitate the process. If you feel the need for more practical advice, read the rest of this chapter, which is all relevant to successful team building.

Dealing with opposition – acting assertively

Assertion is not the same as aggression. Assertiveness has been defined as a quality demonstrated by individuals who know how they feel and what they want, take definite and clear action to express their views, refuse to be side-tracked, and who ensure others know where they stand.

- An aggressive person seeks dominance: aggressiveness involves attempts to intimidate others and violate their rights.
- An assertive person exercises a right to express a viewpoint and have it fully heard while respecting the rights of others.

One characteristic of clinical work is fragmentation and fluctuation in work rate. An essential skill needed by doctors, in the protection of their work routines, is the ability to prevent others from unnecessary, disruptive interference. This is a common cause of frustration and impairs performance, particularly for those who hold supervisory responsibilities, no matter how small. Working in teams means managing your work with others. Maintaining good working relationships while avoiding exploitation of goodwill can be difficult. Achieving and maintaining a satisfactory level of independence, while still contributing fully to co-operative tasks, requires a high level of social and group-working skills. Among these is the ability to act assertively when required – to decline taking on further demands when already fully loaded.

There are many reasons why you may find it hard to say 'No' even to unreasonable demands that are made of you. The more obvious reasons are around the difficulty of deciding what tasks should, or should not, be a part of your role. Equally, you may be unable to define what is a reasonable workload. Job descriptions can help, but are rarely sufficiently detailed to remove all uncertainty, and constant changes in detail mean they are seldom kept up to date.

It is difficult to maintain good relationships with colleagues without constantly succumbing to their demands. Unhealthy conflict can arise if we appear to be negative in our responses. It is suggested that, in addition to 'fight or flight' responses to conflict, we have been conditioned by our parents to respond passively and 'turn the other cheek'. Harris (1970) described the impact of early life experiences on our later behaviours. In developing the concept of transactional analysis, he outlines the nature of 'life scripts'. These are responses we learn early in life that help to shape our view of ourselves and hence our behaviour when responding to others. Harris suggests that our behaviour is shaped by our use of life data which are derived from early experience of key relationships. Hence, interactions with others are shaped by our tendency to respond from the 'parent', 'adult' or 'child' within us. Since the interaction is two-sided, the response we give is frequently drawn out by the type of initial message we receive. Parental instructions, which are likely to be judgemental and directive, tend to bring out the child in us, and vice versa. Overriding the tendency to behave in this pre-determined manner is difficult. It requires the learning of new ways of reacting to requests and demands on our time.

The first and most basic requirement we have in developing the ability to act assertively is to recognise the assertive rights of human beings. Here are a few of these:

- to judge your own behaviour, thoughts and emotions, and to take responsibility for their initiation and consequences upon yourself
- to offer no reasons or excuses to justify your behaviour
- to make mistakes and be responsible for them
- to be treated with respect as an intelligent, capable and equal human being
- to express your feelings.

Assertive behaviour is neither aggressive nor passive. It does not infringe the assertive rights of others. It allows each party to depart with their own self-respect intact. Ideally, it should leave each party feeling 'OK'. It is usually concerned with helping individuals to acquire what is rightfully theirs, to say 'No' to what they do not want or enable them to handle criticism.

Most people recognise their own need to behave assertively when they reflect on their inability to refuse requests for assistance from colleagues, friends or family members, realising they place unreasonable demands on their time or other resources. The early life conditioning referred to above is the most common reason for this weakness. Having convinced ourselves that we have a right to say 'No', the next task is to learn how to say it assertively.

There are two sides to saying 'No'. The first is to recognise how simple it is to find the word. It helps to practise saying it without apologising excessively or making complicated excuses. The dominant reason for experiencing difficulty in refusing an invitation or request is the feeling of guilt that results. The rights referred to above will (if remembered) help to assuage the guilt. So also will the continued use of the skill, so it feels normal. A refusal to a request is not a rejection of the person making the request. Once this fact has been learned the process will become much easier to use. The other side is to develop the skill of saying 'No' using a tone which is at once friendly but firm. The way in which we look and express ourselves has a greater impact on the communication than the words we use.

Sometimes people with whom we deal are persistent in their demands. This increases the challenge, but need not create a problem. The key to success is calm repetition. This is sometimes referred to as the 'broken record'. It enables you to feel comfortable in avoiding manipulative verbal side-traps, argumentative baiting and irrelevant logic. Simply keep repeating your requirement or refusal in a calm and assertive manner until the other person accepts it.

Handling manipulative criticism can also cause difficulty. Assertive responses encompass a range of options. The first is to calmly acknowledge to the critic that there may be some truth in the criticism, yet leave yourself with the right to determine what you will do about it. A stage beyond this is to agree strongly with hostile or constructive criticism as it is given, accepting your faults without resorting to denial. This has the effect of reducing your critic's anger or hostility without making you feel anxious or defensive. There is still no need to apologise if you do not wish to do so.

If it does not weaken your position or threaten your self-respect it is acceptable to seek a workable compromise with the other person. This involves recognising that a 'win-win' situation can be achieved by agreeing to concede something of your own position, while retaining your right to protect your own needs.

The objective of assertive behaviour is not to win all your conflicts at the expense of someone else. It is, rather, to maintain your own position and protect your own rights as a person while dealing effectively with the demands of others around you. It should always be your aim to respect the equivalent rights of others. It is this that differentiates assertive from aggressive behaviour.

Skills of assertion can be identified and learned, increasing the ability to make a positive impact on others – a key factor for those in leadership roles. So let us consider some guidelines for exercising assertion in the face of the opposition.

- Build your argument step by step thus ensuring people have the opportunity to understand your position.
- Say what you need from others as people need to know how they fit into larger plans.
- Communicate in language that others understand to ensure you convey messages in ways that make sense to the listeners.
- Avoid confused emotions. If you are angry, hurt or emotionally upset others are more likely to respond to your feelings than your message. This can confuse the issues.
- Make it simple. People often lose the strength of their argument by excessive complexity or by dealing with several issues at once.
- Work towards resolving the questions and concerns of others. This may involve continuing to put your message across until you are satisfied a resolution can be achieved.
- Do not put yourself down. If something is important to you let others know where you stand.
- Watch out for 'flak'; others may try to divert you from your message. You may feel under pressure. Acknowledge their views but always return to your position.
- Error does not weaken. We all make mistakes and errors should not make you feel inadequate. A sense of inadequacy will undermine your position.

People who face conflict assertively are said to:

- be open about their objectives
- establish the other person's objectives
- search for common ground
- state their case clearly
- understand the other person's case
- produce ideas to solve differences
- build on and add to the other person's ideas
- summarise to check understanding and agreement.

Action

Reflect on your own situation in putting forward sensitive issues to others or being asked to undertake extra jobs. For example, changes in rotas, changes in routine work, dealing with extra cases, patients added to out-patient lists and having to cover for others at short notice.

How do you rate according to the above guidelines?

Resolving conflict in work groups

Our research confirmed the importance doctors attach to the effective working of the teams to which they belong. An occasional consequence of the pressure medical practitioners are subjected to is the generation of tension and conflict within the team. This section helps to identify your approach to the handling of conflict.

Conflict handling style

What is your preferred style when faced with conflict?

Conflict style inventory

Derived from: Pfeiffer and Goodstein (1982) (*see* Related reading, p. 53).

Instructions

Choose a single frame of reference for answering all 15 items (e.g. work-related, family or social conflicts) and keep that frame of reference in mind when answering all items.

Allocate ten points among the four alternative answers given for each of the 15 items below. For example, **when the people I organise become involved in a personal conflict, I would usually . . .**

intervene to settle the dispute.	call a meeting to talk over the problem.	offer to help if I can.	ignore the problem.
3	6	1	0
_____	_____	_____	_____

Be sure that your answers add up to ten.

1 **When someone I care about is actively hostile toward me (i.e. threatening, shouting, abusive, etc.) I tend to . . .**

respond in a hostile manner.	try to persuade the person to give up his/her actively hostile behaviour.	stay and listen as long as possible.	walk away.
_____	_____	_____	_____

2 **When someone who is relatively unimportant to me is actively hostile toward me (i.e. yelling, threatening, abusive, etc.) I tend to . . .**

respond in a hostile manner.	try to persuade the person to give up his/her actively hostile behaviour.	stay and listen as long as possible.	walk away.
_____	_____	_____	_____

3 **When I observe people in conflicts in which anger, threats, hostility and strong opinions are present I tend to . . .**

become involved and take a position.	attempt to mediate.	observe to see what happens.	leave as quickly as possible.
_____	_____	_____	_____

4 **When I perceive another person as meeting his/her needs at my expense I am apt to . . .**

work to do anything I can to change that person.	rely on persuasion and facts when attempting to have that person change.	work hard at changing how I relate to that person.	accept the situation as it is.
_____	_____	_____	_____

5 When involved in an interpersonal dispute my general pattern is to . . .

draw the other person into seeing the problem as I do.	examine the issues between us as logically as possible.	look hard for a workable compromise.	let time take its course and let the problem work itself out.
_____	_____	_____	_____

6 The quality that I value the most in dealing with conflict would be . . .

emotional strength and security.	intelligence.	love and openness.	patience.
_____	_____	_____	_____

7 Following a serious altercation with someone I care for deeply I . . .

strongly desire to go back and settle things my way.	want to go back and work it out whatever give and take is necessary.	worry about it a lot but not plan to initiate further contact.	let it lie and not plan to initiate further contact.
_____	_____	_____	_____

8 When I see a serious conflict developing between two people I care about I tend to . . .

express my disappointment that this had to happen.	attempt to persuade them to resolve their differences.	watch to see what develops.	leave the scene.
_____	_____	_____	_____

9 When I see a serious conflict developing between two people who are relatively unimportant to me I tend to . . .

express my disappointment that this had to happen.	attempt to persuade them to resolve their differences.	watch to see what develops.	leave the scene.
_____	_____	_____	_____

10 The feedback I receive from most people about how I behave when faced with conflict and opposition indicates that I . . .

try hard to get my way.	try to work out differences cooperatively.	am easygoing and take a soft or conciliatory position.	usually avoid the conflict.
_____	_____	_____	_____

11 When communicating with someone with whom I am having a serious conflict I . . .

try to overpower the other person with my speech.	talk a little bit more than I listen (feeding back words and feelings).	am an active listener (agreeing and apologising).	am a passive listener.
_____	_____	_____	_____

12 When involved in an unpleasant conflict I . . .

use humour with the other party.	make an occasional quip or joke about the situation or the relationship.	relate humour only to myself.	suppress all attempts at humour.
_____	_____	_____	_____

13 When someone does something that irritates me (e.g. smokes in a non-smoking area or crowds in line in front of me) my tendency in communicating with the offending person is to . . .

use strong, direct language and tell the person to stop.	try to persuade the person to stop.	talk gently and tell the person what my feelings are.	say and do nothing.
_____	_____	_____	_____

14 When someone does something that irritates me (e.g. smokes in a non-smoking area or crowds in line in front of me) my tendency in communicating with the offending person is to . . .

stand close and make physical contact.	use my hands and body to illustrate my points.	stand close to the person without touching him or her.	stand back and keep my hands to myself.
_____	_____	_____	_____

15 When someone does something that irritates me (e.g. smokes in a non-smoking area or queue-jumps in front of me) my tendency in communicating with the offending person is to . . .

insist that the person look me in the eye.	look the person directly in the eye and maintain eye contact.	maintain intermittent eye contact.	avoid looking directly at the person.
_____	_____	_____	_____

Scoring and interpretation

Instructions

When you have completed all 15 items, add your scores vertically, resulting in four column totals. Put these on the blanks below.

TOTALS =

_____	_____	_____	_____
Column 1	**Column 2**	**Column 3**	**Column 4**

Column 1 – Aggressive/Confrontive

High scores indicate a tendency to 'taking the bull by the horns' and a strong need to control situations and/or people. Those who use this style are often directive and judgemental.

Column 2 – Assertive/Persuasive

High scores indicate a tendency to stand up for oneself without being pushy, a proactive approach to conflict and a willingness to collaborate. People who use this style depend heavily on their verbal skills.

Column 3 – Observant/Introspective

High scores indicate a tendency to observe others and examine oneself analytically in response to conflict situations, as well as a need to adopt counselling and listening models of behaviour. Those who use this style are likely to be cooperative, even conciliatory.

Column 4 – Avoiding/Reactive

High scores indicate a tendency toward passivity or withdrawal in conflict situations and a need to avoid confrontation. Those who use this style are usually accepting and patient, often suppressing their strong feelings.

Now total your scores for Columns 1 and 2 and Columns 3 and 4.

Column 1 + Column 2 = Score A; Column 3 + Column 4 = Score B.

If Score A is significantly higher than Score B (25 points or more), it may indicate a tendency toward aggressive/assertive conflict management. A significantly higher B score signals a more conciliatory approach.

Conflict is certain to occur from time to time when people work closely together, especially if their work sometimes involves making difficult decisions together. Understanding how you normally react to conflict is the first stage in developing strategies for dealing with it in a way which suits your personality, while achieving the best results in your work. Colleagues respond differently according to a wide variety of factors, some of which might involve their current life pressures, whereas others are more concerned with their continuing view of themselves and others. Getting to know the things that affect other individuals can be as important as knowing yourself.

Handling conflict can, and often does, give rise to anger on either or both sides. We all feel anger sometimes and see it in others. But how can we personally handle both our and other's anger?

Dealing with your own anger

The earlier you tackle it the better; do not kid yourself that something is not worth the hassle, but if you have had a few drinks wait until the effect has worn off. You can release some of your physical tension by exercise even if it is only hitting a cushion. Then coolly analyse the situation and decide what you are going to say to address it.

You can be positive and direct but don't make it personal. Avoid saying the person made you angry but rather that you felt threatened. Acknowledge some responsibility, perhaps for not saying something earlier, but avoid self put-downs, invitations to retaliatory criticism and don't bring up past grievances. Don't stereotype, moralise or bring in third parties. Remember to:

- criticise the behaviour not the person
- be specific and realistic in any request
- avoid humour
- use assertive language.

Dealing with anger from someone else

Sometimes you will find yourself having to handle an angry colleague, patient or patient's relative. Try to remember how you have felt when you were angry, and remember that it was not easy to be rational. The following points will help.

- Try to be on a level with the other person – if you are looking down on them they may feel more threatened.
- Keep your own voice as level as possible – try to communicate calm through the way you speak to the person.

- Allow them plenty of personal space as getting too close may also make them feel threatened.
- Acknowledge the other's feelings with an empathic statement. The other person, then realising that you understand, will no longer have to prove their anger.
- Indicate you are listening by reflective listening and repeating back a summary of what is being said.
- Avoid questioning an angry person.
- If you are in a closed space or room, check you are well positioned for leaving quickly, or at least ensure that a large piece of furniture separates you from the complainant!

Use simple assertiveness techniques (*see* p. 36 on assertiveness) such as the 'broken record' to express yourself calmly and persistently. An angry person often leaps from topic to topic. These points are also covered in handling patient complaints, p. 115.

Delegation

You may well feel that as a SpR you have little need of delegation skills. But have you considered how you make the best of opportunities to work with other SpRs, SHOs, PRHOs, medical students, nurses, technicians, phlebotomists, physiotherapists, pharmacists, auxiliaries, receptionists, secretaries, medical record clerks, audit assistants and others?

Delegation is not just about getting others to do the unpleasant, dirty, tedious or boring jobs that you do not want to do. It is also about sharing out the interesting things. You have a responsibility to help others, including your junior colleagues, to develop them and increase their experience. This will not happen unless you take positive steps to make it happen. You may not think this too important now, but the more senior you become, the more you will need to delegate. You cannot do everything yourself. When you become a consultant you will have a great need to be skilful at delegation.

Good time management involves making the most effective use of all staff resources, including your own. Tasks that can be carried out satisfactorily by others listed in the examples above should not necessarily be routinely undertaken by you. The complex nature of healthcare demands specialist knowledge and skills. Rapid change, brought on by technological development, has increased the complexity of the work of doctors. It is impossible for an individual to carry all the knowledge and skills necessary to ensure effective performance of the unit. Delegation is not just about telling others to perform particular tasks. It provides a mechanism for controlled sharing of the workload.

Delegation is achieving results by enabling and motivating others who are usually more junior to you, to carry out tasks (for which you are ultimately accountable) to an accepted, agreed level of competence. The concept of delegation is simple. The practice is rather different and involves high levels of skill and understanding. Delegation is usually interpreted to mean passing down authority and responsibility to others at a more junior level. It is also possible to 'delegate laterally' to other SpRs and colleagues, for example when a surgical SpR hands over the responsibility for preparing a case for theatre or when a medical SpR hands over responsibility for a severe haematemesis to a surgeon. Even upward delegation may take place when, for example, an SHO is called to an emergency elsewhere in the hospital. The SpR may agree to continue with the ward round or the theatre case they were carrying out together.

Authority and responsibility

Authority and responsibility go together. Authority is the power and the right to take appropriate action in a given situation. Responsibility is an individual's 'answerability' for the successful accomplishment of a task. It would be unreasonable to delegate responsibility for an activity without giving the person authority to act. For example, if the ward phoned theatre to ask an anaesthetic SpR for analgesia (administered in a previous case but not written up) and the SpR sent the anaesthetic SHO to write up the prescription, it would be unreasonable to expect the SHO to bring the treatment sheet back to be written up by the SpR. Similarly, if a person is given authority, they should be held responsible for the outcome. If the SHO writes up the wrong dose or drug, they are responsible for that error. This does not mean a doctor can delegate *ultimate* responsibility. If the SHO had been a PRHO and it was their first day, it might be considered unreasonable to delegate that task to them. Or maybe the surgical SpR is operating and the list is running late. It is suggested that the last case, to be performed under local anaesthesia, is carried out in a now empty theatre by another member of the team. If the SHO is delegated the task by the SpR it would be unreasonable to expect them to constantly check every step with the SpR before operating. Equally, if that person is given authority, they should be held responsible for outcomes. If the SHO does the wrong operation, the SHO is responsible for that error. If, on the other hand, the SHO had no experience of the procedure, it would be considered unreasonable to delegate the task to them. You should be able to think of other examples within your own specialty.

The role is to delegate effectively and give support, encouragement and reasonable protection to staff. A doctor remains accountable for all the activities, whether medical or managerial, within his or her control.

Performance evaluation

Evaluation of performance and recognition of achievement are additional factors in the process of delegation. Effective control should mean you check on the satisfactory completion of the delegated task and feedback given to the successful SHO.

Difficulties arise largely as a result of the emotional link we have with our own work. We worry that another person might not do it as well as we would, or worse, they might show us up by being much better at it! It is often easier to do it yourself than explain to someone else how to do it. Sometimes we feel uncomfortable about asking others because they are too busy or the task is unpleasant. There is the need to show trust in our juniors so they can develop. Tension sometimes arises because of the relationship which inevitably exists in the 'trust/control relationship'. The amount of control we retain reduces with any increase in trust we demonstrate in the person to whom we delegate.

Motivation

We have already discussed in some detail on p. 31 what motivates people, when we discussed leadership, but it might be useful to repeat the key factors, as understanding how to motivate people is fundamental to your success in delegation. The performance of any individual in the conduct of their work is likely to be dependent on three variables.

- The *ability* to complete the task satisfactorily – a combination of aptitude and training.
- The equipment and facilities for the job must be available; they must have the *opportunity*.
- They must be *motivated* to complete the task.

Much has been written in management literature on the subject of motivation. Most general management textbooks have at least one chapter on the subject.

On p. 29 we also discussed how good leaders are able to understand what motivates the staff and act accordingly in order to get the best from them.

Guidelines for successful delegation

Doctors work in teams made up of individuals who possess a complex range of skills and are often sensitive with regard to their status in the team. If good results are to be achieved, successful delegation requires careful thought and the exercise of skill in dealing with individuals.

Action

Identify a task you perform which you could ask a colleague or junior to do instead of you. It should be a task you consider to be important but not unsafe to allow others to undertake.

- Identify a person to whom you could delegate the task. Choose the right person, taking into account ability, personality and potential.
- Consult with the individual before finally deciding the extent of the delegated task.
- Delegate the *whole* task, not parts that do not carry significant responsibility.
- Clarify the purpose, limits and outcomes or expected results of the task.
- Instruct them on the best methods and give clear guidance on what they should do if they need help.
- Be prepared to delegate enjoyable tasks as well as those which no one wants. You will motivate people that way.
- Trust the person to get on with the task and allow them to decide when they need help, subject to agreed monitoring arrangements.
- Review their performance after a reasonable time has passed.
- Review your own performance. Note any improvement in the way in which you are able to carry out your core responsibilities.

The politics of influencing outcomes

Organisational relationships in hospitals are complex and involve most doctors in membership of a wide range of subgroups. Formal structures sometimes exist as diagrams showing divisions, directorates and so on, but these only partly describe the reality of groups or coalitions to which doctors (and others) relate or belong.

There are two broad categories of group – formal and informal. Sometimes informal groups, although not recognised in the formal structure of the hospital, have a very powerful influence on events.

One of the most valuable interpersonal skills is the ability to influence others. It can be used across hierarchical boundaries as well as in traditional managerial roles. Influence rests on the ability to use various forms of power. Usually there are said to be five sources of power. Their suitability in exerting influence is affected by both access to them and current circumstances. They are related to:

Position in the organisation: authority is vested in a post enabling people in more senior positions to influence subordinates.

Expertise held by the post-holder: others will usually defer to the person who (they perceive) has expert knowledge.

Control over *resources*: sometimes people have power well beyond their status in an organisation because they control access to resources others need. Information may be regarded as a resource and control over information is sometimes used by relatively junior employees to exert influence over others.

Personal charm or *charisma*: there are a few people we meet who can influence others without appearing to have special powers other than their natural ability to lead.

Coercion: often exerted through an implied threat that induces fear in those who can be influenced by the possible outcome. Not usually regarded as an attractive option, it is sometimes used to achieve change in the face of resistance from those affected by the change.

Insight into the sources of power and those who control them can be a useful tool. Power and influence can sometimes be acquired by aligning with those who hold power. At other times it may be wise to avoid them.

Action

Write your name in the centre of an A4 sheet. Now write in the names and/or job titles of all those with whom you interact in your work and work-related activities. Include social contacts, particularly those who have more influence in your organisation than you.

Group into formal contacts by drawing lines between connected names. Some names or titles are likely to be part of your *informal* network. Circle these and list them separately. Consider whether any of these are particularly influential in the context of the organisation. How could they help you to achieve your personal goals? How do you relate to them at present? Could you do more to employ their strengths on your own behalf?

What sources of power do you currently exploit?

Which others could you exploit?

Which do you encourage those working with or for you to develop?

Handling stress

Most professionals become familiar with the concept of work overload at some stage in their careers. For many the effects can be recognised in the deterioration of their capacity for taking on new challenges and maintenance of normal lifestyle and family relationships. A less obvious side effect is the impact uneven work patterns can have on health. Stress is often blamed as the instrument which directs the ill effects. It has been described as a trigger for a multitude of physical and mental disorders, including heart disease and cancer. Most authors prefer to see stress as describing a spectrum of states of mind, which includes stress as a positive, as well as negative, concept. Thus, it may be described as a demand made on the adaptive capacities of the mind and body. It is only when demand becomes more than the mind and body can handle that its effects become undesirable. Before this stage, it can act as a spur to greater achievement and satisfaction at work.

In order to understand the stresses in our lives we need to assess the external demands made on us (and that we make on ourselves) and our own capacity for handling that stress. People vary widely in their personal capacity for dealing with work overload. What appears as a major problem to one person may be an exciting challenge to another.

Personality

Personalities and their approach to work-related stress have been assessed according to type. Complete the following questionnaire. Answer each question 'yes' or 'no'.

1 Do you characteristically do several things at once (e.g. telephoning, reading your post and jotting notes on a pad)?
2 Do you feel guilty when relaxing, as if there is always something else you should be doing?
3 Are you quickly bored when other people are talking? Do you find yourself wanting to interrupt or hurry them up?
4 Do you try to steer conversation towards your own interests, instead of wanting to hear those of others?
5 Are you usually anxious to finish each of your tasks so you can get on to the next?
6 Are you unobservant when it comes to anything that is not immediately connected with what you are actually doing?
7 Do you prefer to have rather than to be (i.e. to experience your possessions rather than to experience yourself)?
8 Do you do most things (e.g. eating, talking and walking) at high speed?
9 Do you find people like yourself, challenging and people who dawdle, infuriating?
10 Are you physically tense and assertive?

11 Are you more interested in winning than in simply taking part and enjoying your-self?
12 Do you find it hard to laugh at yourself?
13 Do you find it hard to delegate?
14 Do you find it almost impossible to attend meetings without speaking up?
15 Do you prefer activity holidays to dreamy, relaxing ones?
16 Do you push those for whom you feel responsible (e.g. children, subordinates or part-ner) to try to achieve your own standards, without showing much interest in what they really want out of life?

It has been suggested that personality types can be divided into those who are driven by ambition and the need to achieve (Type A) and those more laid-back people for whom life is a series of experiences which may be outside their control, but can be nonetheless enjoyable (Type B). People with extreme Type A personalities will have answered 'yes' to all 16 questions above. If you have responded positively to 12 or more of the questions, then you are likely to have significant Type A tendencies. Type A people like deadlines and pressures, are impatient to move on to new challenges and can be intolerant of the failure of others to measure up to their own standards of commitment. Unfortunately, this approach to life can lead to Type As drawing more upon themselves than they can reasonably cope with, finding they have fewer coping mechanisms as the pressure rises to breaking point.

Lifestyle

Maintenance of a balanced lifestyle, in which sport, leisure and family pursuits are given equal place with work, is seen as an essential prerequisite for holding on to healthy stress levels. This helps to ensure that the volume and nature of the workload does not outpace the individual's capacity for managing the work. This is usually easier said than done in modern working environments, where pressure to absorb increasing demand is often linked to organisational survival. Techniques of time management, as described in Chapter 1, can be used to begin the process of re-dressing the balance between work and leisure activities.

Another complementary approach is to increase the capacity of individuals for coping with high levels of stress. Changing lifestyle is not easy, but can be managed, especially if the consequences of failure to do so are taken into account. People with Type A personalities will be able to recognise the kinds of things that can be done to reduce the risk of stress. Paradoxically, they can be most effective in implementing change programmes to improve themselves. Finding and developing non-work interests that provide an antidote to overwork can make a good start to the process. Competitive sports, such as golf or sailing, can help to improve physical fitness and enable escape from work pressure for significant periods of time. Learning to delegate, which is discussed earlier in this chapter, is also vitally important for people with Type A personalities.

Relaxation

Some writers on stress management advocate the use of relaxation and meditation techniques. These range from undertaking simple physical exercises to the acquisition of understanding of Eastern philosophies and habits of mind. They do not work for everyone. It has been argued that regular meditation, even for only a few minutes each day, builds the ability to concentrate and handle emotions, and aids physical relaxation. Some people find it difficult to acquire the mental discipline associated with such an approach, although simple physical relaxation techniques are within the scope of the majority. A wide range of books on stress management and relaxation techniques is available. Many replicate the same basic approach.

An example of advice on meditative technique is shown below. Try it, as it may be right for you. Certain personalities will feel unhappy with this type of approach. It requires practice to become competent so persevere before deciding whether it works for you or not. Perhaps try it only for five minutes the first few times, and rise to ten or more after a week or so.

- Choose a suitable room or place where you are guaranteed peace and quiet, free from interruption. Sit in a comfortable, upright chair. Keep your body upright throughout. It may help to imagine that your head is held up by a connection with the ceiling above you. Allow your muscles to relax as much as possible while still keeping an upright posture. Close your eyes.
- Remaining as calm as possible, start to focus on your breathing. You will find it helps to concentrate on either your nostrils or your abdomen, but not on both. Count one for each breath as you finish breathing out. Count up to ten, then down again until you reach one. Keep repeating this process.
- As thoughts arise, allow them to drift without paying attention to them. Do not try to drive them away. Concentrate on your breathing. Allow other thoughts to come and go without hindrance.
- After the meditation session is over, rise slowly from your chair. Try to maintain the poised awareness you experienced while meditating. Apply the same approach to thinking about the sights and sounds around you as you go about your everyday activities.

This approach will not remove the source of stress. In serious situations radical life change may be necessary, such as a change of career direction. Meditation and other techniques are, arguably, a way of managing stress, rather than allowing it to manage us.

Learning to handle stress

Changing the way we think about our lives is difficult. It has been suggested that the following characteristics are found in those who handle stress most effectively.

- They shelve problems until they are capable of dealing with them. They do not dwell on issues with which they cannot cope.
- They deliberately relax after coping with highly demanding and stressful tasks, usually by undertaking contrasting activities.
- They take a wider view of situations and do not become bogged down in detail.
- They control the build up and pace of stressful situations via planning and intervening to prevent themselves from becoming swamped.
- They are prepared to confront difficulties or unpleasant issues.
- They know their own capacity and do not permit themselves to become overwhelmed by events.
- They can cope with being unpopular.
- They do not commit themselves to very tight deadlines which are unlikely to be met.
- They actively limit their involvement in work in order to maintain a balanced lifestyle.

The previous section on stress management is intended to provide an insight into the issues. It does not deal with the responsibility that those supervising the work of others have in ensuring safe and realistic work programmes for them.

Related reading

Beels C, Hopson B and Scally M (1992) *Assertiveness: a positive process*. Lifeskills Communications Ltd, London.

Fontana D (1989) *Managing Stress*. British Psychological Society/Routledge, London.

Francis D and Woodcock M (1996) *The New Unblocked Manager*. Gower, London.

Harris TA (1970) *I'm OK, You're OK*. Pan, London.

Lindenfield G (1998) *Managing Anger*. Thorsons, London.

Mullins LJ (1998) *Management and Organisational Behaviour* (5e). Financial Times, Prentice Hall, London.

Pfeiffer JW and Goodstein LD (eds) (1982) *The 1982 Annual for Facilitators, Trainers, and Consultants*. University Associates, San Diego, CA.

Pfeiffer JW and Jones JE (eds) (1974) *A Handbook of Structured Experiences in Human Relations Training*, vol 1 (revised). University Associates, San Diego, CA.

Quick TL (1992) *Successful Team Building*. Amacom, New York.

Smith MJ (1975) *When I Say No I Feel Guilty*. Bantam, London.

Tichy NM and Devanna MA (1986) *The Transformational Leader*. John Wiley, New York.

3

Communicating effectively

The aim of this chapter is to provide you with a foundation on which to develop your written and face-to-face communication skills.

The chapter also covers the role of information in the NHS and the use of information technology in clinical medicine and training.

Effective writing

Communication seems easy enough when we talk to people face to face. Yet mysteriously, those who can charm an audience at a party, when armed with a word processor, use convoluted constructions and obscure words that baffle a reader before the second full stop. Effective writing is the creative use of words in an easily readable form which sends a message from one person to another, accurately and completely.

According to Tim Albert, Visiting Fellow in medical writing at Southampton Medical School, on whose work this information is based, one of the most misleading and pretentious phrases used by scientists is 'in the literature'. The kind of writing dealt with here has nothing to do with pure literature, which is generally written by enthusiasts for themselves, and only rarely considered good enough to be published and shared with others. The kind of writing discussed here is more functional and concerned mainly with putting messages across, not just out.

Medical schools encourage young men and women to reject 'real' English in favour of the particular language of medicine. This is acceptable when communicating with other doctors. When communicating with other people it becomes meaningless gibberish. Further traps await. Medicine, like all other professions, is highly competitive. Writing is in black and white. Those who have to commit themselves take great care not to offend their peers and, if possible, try to impress upon them the author's grasp of the subject. This is often an effective way of ensuring that the message fails to get through.

The all-important principle is to write with your readers' interests in mind at all times. This principle allows for all other rules to be broken. For instance, if the reader will understand better when you split an infinitive, then you should split one. If the reader has limited knowledge you should simplify. If the reader needs to come away with a vague or softened message, then you should wheel out your euphemisms. Apart from our single principle, there are no absolute, hard-and-fast rules.

The process of writing

Forward planning is helpful. Avoid huge undertakings like 'writing a paper' or 'doing a report'. Break these down into small units, such as 'five possible topics for an article' or the 'headings' for the report.

You do not need to be seated at a desk to do this. As Klauser (1987) points out in her excellent book on the process of writing, 'ruminating time' is an essential part of the writing process. The thought you invest at the beginning pays dividends. The structure and style of a report differs depending on whether it is written for a lay reader or doctor. Writing too much is not a sign that the writer is well informed, but rather that he or she has failed to make basic decisions on what is really important for the audience. And remember your deadline. It should be realistic, allowing ample time for revisions and changes.

The best start, as Klauser suggests, is 'mind-mapping'. This involves writing down on a clean sheet of paper the elements of the theme. Then start jotting down questions and thoughts that you will need to deal with, taking them out like the branches of a tree. This technique is explained by Buzan (1989) (*see* Chapter 1, Related reading).

Most writers suggest that you write a first draft of the whole piece in one go. Once you have finished this, put it away for a few days (or at least overnight). When you return to it, relatively fresh, you can start the real work. Leave it for as long as possible, then start revising.

Active or passive?

There is a common argument that professional people should not use the first person. The passive has three disadvantages. It requires more words, it becomes less vigorous and the writer often fails to state who actually performed the action.

We are indebted to Tim Albert for the following example:

- **Passive**

  'The questionnaires were administered and the results were subsequently analysed. It was discovered after analysis that action was indicated.'

- **Active**

  The passive statement above could mean either of the following alternatives:

  'Trained interviewers administered the questionnaires and processed the results. I analysed the figures and concluded that the Director of Public Health had a problem.'

  'A work experience student administered the questionnaire and her boyfriend used his computer to process the results. They looked at some of the comments and decided to send them to the *News of the World*.'

The passive does have a place. It is useful when the object of an action is more important than the subject or when causality has yet to be established. And it is also useful when a writer, quite deliberately or for political reasons, wishes to make things unclear. Writing in the active, on the other hand, is one of the most effective ways of improving dense prose. As Gowers (1986), one of the leading authorities on effective style, remarks dryly: 'Overuse of the passive may render a sentence impenetrable'.

General reports

There are frequently 'local' rules which should be followed. These are determined by custom and practice within an organisation or profession. The following are general guidelines which can be adapted to the expectations of the population within which your report will be circulated.

Define the brief carefully and pay attention to the real audience. Avoid technical words and jargon. Study other reports. Pay particular attention to the structure. You will usually have headings and subheadings. Within each of these sections the usual guidelines apply. Use the conclusion to put across the message you wish to stay in the reader's mind. In addition, give a summary, so that busy readers can at least have a quick overview.

Initially we will deal with the general framework or layout for writing a report. This might be a report of an incident or event, an audit report or a medico-legal report. There is no right and wrong way – different people have different views and ideas – but some general principles emerge.

A typical general report

Title page – includes the title and date of the report and the author's name.

Contents page – lists all the main sections and subsections of the report and the pages on which they appear.

Acknowledgements – it is common practice to name and thank sources of help and advice.

Aims and objectives/Terms of reference – defines as precisely as possible the purpose for which the report has been prepared and the limits placed on it. Each of these possible section headings has a different meaning: aims are broad statements of intent; objectives are usually stated as 'measurable' outcomes; terms of reference describe precisely the limits placed on the report as well as its aims or objectives.

Abstract or summary – sometimes placed as the front page of the document, this serves to inform the reader of the essence of the whole report in a few words.

Summary of conclusions/Recommendations – either or both may be presented at the front end of the report. This is dependent on local practice and the nature of the report objectives. They can be presented in tabular or bulleted form and should be as brief and simple as possible.

Introduction – describes (briefly) the background to the report, the scope and the limitations of the report. The reader should be clear about why the report has been written and, therefore, why it should be worth reading.

Methods and/or methodology – often used to describe the same thing, these two words have different meanings. Methods describe the way data were collected. The reasons for selecting one method rather than another should be explained. Methodology requires more fundamental consideration and explanation. Put simply, it is the way the data are used to obtain results and conclusions. It describes an approach to research. Remember you do not take children to the zoology to see the animals.

Results or findings – outcomes and information presented in some sort of logical sequence, dealing perhaps with one area at a time by dividing into three or four further sections. You may include some discussion or opinion in this section but distinguish between fact and opinion. We have already alluded to the impersonal or personal style of writing. In the past, report writing was very much an impersonal or third-person approach. Indeed many journals will still not consider any other format. There is now a clear move to greater acceptance of the personal approach to writing thoughts and opinions, certainly as you must be willing to stand by what you write.

The placing of tables, diagrams and graphs is a matter of personal choice. This can be a good place to include them if they help to clarify the message within the body of the report. If there is too much information, but you believe the reader should be given an opportunity to see it, then put it into an appendix. Always remember the guiding principle – write with the readers' interests in mind at all times.

Conclusions – should emerge from the results and therefore may be simply cross-referenced to previous sections so that the reader can easily follow the author's arguments. Conclusions should also only be within the scope of the terms of reference. Avoid introducing something new into the conclusions which has not been explained previously.

Recommendations – should flow naturally from the report and its conclusions and again cross-referencing enables both author and reader to follow the flow of logic. It is worth considering the 'political' implications of your recommendations which would require action by others. Perhaps time spent preparing the ground before the report is published would be time well spent.

Bibliography – sometimes included at this stage, or as an appendix, if the report needs one. References may be placed here as an alternative to within the text.

Appendices – start each appendix on a separate page. This section includes graphs, diagrams, charts, statistics, schedules, calculations, plans and source data. Define terms and explain terminology which may be unfamiliar to the target audience.

Memos and letters

The most appropriate structure is known as the 'inverted triangle'. Put the important part – the payoff for the reader – in the first sentence. The first few words should not be boring, as in: 'I am in receipt of your letter' or 'The car-parking working party of the senior management group...'. Some people expect a welcoming cough, such as: 'Thank you for your letter' or 'It was good to meet you the other day'. This reinforces our main principle: the interests of the reader are paramount.

Medico-legal reports

At some point in your career, particularly if you work in a specialty dealing with trauma cases, solicitors may request you provide a medical report. You normally have no obligation to write this and may wish to hand it on to a colleague, perhaps someone more senior. As you progress in seniority and acquire more experience you will probably want to write these yourself, particularly as they carry a fee. The size of that fee will depend on the complexity of the case and the time and work involved, but the BMA publishes guidelines on such fees and you can always discuss and compare your experience with colleagues locally.

You will normally be asked to address a particular issue. This is your 'remit'. Some will require examination of the patient. Issues you may need to address will include:

- condition
- prognosis
- negligence
- causation.

The medical evidence provided by your report must comply with the requirements of Civil Justice Rules (1998). We recommend, therefore, that before preparing and writing any medico-legal report you obtain a copy of the notes and Part 35 of the Civil Procedure Rules (1998) and the Supplementary Practice Directions.

Try to be proactive with the lawyer who requests the report. Ask questions until you are confident you understand clearly what is being requested. You will need the following:

- hospital records
- x-rays and scans
- general practitioner records
- previous reports
- patient's statement, if appropriate (personal injury cases).

Hospitals usually charge for these, so it is normal practice for the solicitor to supply them, or at least copies. Well-organised law firms will supply them in chronological order and paginated.

Structuring a medico-legal report

Type with double space and wide margins. The style and layout can vary, although it is largely determined by the Civil Procedure Rules (1998). It is also influenced by the writer and partly by the needs of the solicitor or barrister. You will be required to state the extent of your contact with the patient, the history, symptoms and other details as relevant. Avoid technical jargon unless you give an explanation. Remember that lawyers are interested in the strengths and weaknesses of the case, particularly the latter. Give the results of examinations and investigations and state your opinion with reasons. Distinguish facts from opinions and recognise your assumptions.

The Civil Procedure Rules (1998) specify that the following requirements must be met. The report must:

- be addressed to the Court

- set out the substance of your instructions
- include details of any literature or other material relied upon
- state who carried out any test or experiment used for the report and whether or not the test or experiment was carried out under your supervision
- give qualifications of any person who carried out any test or experiment
- summarise any range of opinions and give reasons for your own opinion
- set out a summary of the conclusions
- state that you understand your duty to the Court and that you have complied with that duty
- set out the statement of truth in the form required
- give details of your qualifications.

Most of the following suggested sections mainly include statements of fact but you need to exercise care with those that require opinion.

Summary
A front page with a summary is usually helpful and might include the identity of the patient, the date of the report, date of injury, the cause, the injuries or at least those relevant to your report, treatment and progress, a summary of your examination findings and, finally, the prognosis.

Section 1   Instructions
Describe the source and substance of your instructions and the documents, literature or other material you have seen.

Section 2   Details of claimant
This identifies the patient together with age, sex, date of birth, and age at the time of report of any accident or illness. It is helpful to include subheadings for marital status, family and social history, occupational details and leisure activities. Include a section for other factors which do not fit neatly into other sections but which need a mention.

Section 3   Previous medical history
You should refer particularly to anything relevant to the present symptoms.

Section 4   Present complaints
List the patient's symptoms as precisely as possible.

Section 5   History of injury

Section 6   Treatment

Section 7   Progress of treatment

Section 8   Present examination

Section 9   Investigations
It is important to identify any test or investigation undertaken, the qualifications of the person who carried it out, and whether it was under your supervision.

Section 10   Opinion
This is the most important section and will require careful thought. How do you distinguish facts and opinions? Here are some suggested definitions:

- *facts* are real and objective
- *feelings* are emotional responses to situations or events
- *values* are derived from norms in society, the organisation and the family
- *opinions* are our personal ideas or explanations about issues, events or situations
- *assumptions* help to make sense of complexity, but should be distinguished from 'facts'.

In civil proceedings, liability and causation have to be demonstrated on a balance of probabilities. In other words, 'more likely than not'. This could mean a 50.1% chance at least. So the key phrase is 'on the balance of probabilities'. This contrasts with criminal cases, in which the level of proof is generally 'beyond reasonable doubt'.

The Civil Procedure Rules (1998) now require that you summarise any range of opinions as well as giving reasons for your own opinion.

Section 11   Period of incapacity from work or normal activity

Section 12   Period of partial incapacity

Section 13   Residual disability

Section 14   Disfigurement

Section 15   Psychological aspects

Section 16   Special needs

Section 17   Recommendations for treatment and rehabilitation

Section 18 Prognosis and long-term considerations

Section 19   Conclusions
This is distinct from your opinions and should set out a summary of your conclusions, based entirely on the information contained within the report.

Section 20   Compliance with Civil Procedure Rules (1998)
Review your report and confirm that you have complied with and understand your duty to the Court.

Section 21   Your qualifications
State your qualifications, current post and relevant experience.

Section 22   Data Protection Act 1985
Indicate whether you are retaining the records on a computerised system.

Review your report

The important features are that the report should be:

- set out in the form required by the Court
- clearly and concisely written
- clearly presented
- clearly structured
- easy to read.

Each page should be numbered, a header or footer with the patient's name is also useful, and the sections should be numbered for easy reference. Sign and date the report it is easy to forget this! Your fee note should be separate from the report and not referred to in the report.

Important reminders for medico-legal reports

- You must comply with the Civil Procedure Rules (1998).
- Avoid partiality – you are acting as an independent expert. Partiality will compromise your opinion.
- Never gloss over weaknesses. Better they are revealed early in a case.
- Do not stray from your area of expertise as you could find yourself challenged later.

Report submission

What happens to your report after submission? It usually goes to the patient who checks that the history is correct. It may then be sent to counsel who will consider it and write comments. There may be a meeting or conference of experts at this stage, depending on the size of the case. Later you may be asked to review what you have written, as legal issues are often not identical to medical issues. There is nothing sinister in this, but you should not write something to which you cannot put your name or are not prepared to defend.

Getting published

Researching

Specific provision is made for those who wish to undertake a period of research during the SpR training programme *(see* Chapter 10 in *A Guide to Specialist Registrar Training* (1998), NHSE, p. 121). Others are expected to develop an understanding of research methodology and are encouraged to undertake research. Research can be enjoyable, but is time-consuming and can be expensive. In some ways it is like detective work, starting with a problem, going through a process of investigation, building up evidence and moving towards conclusions. The sense of achievement in new discovery can be tremendous, but beyond this personal satisfaction it could be argued that all professional practice should be research-based and research-validated, and all professional doctors have a responsibility to contribute to the process.

Keeping up with the literature

With so many published journals how do you keep up-to-date with the literature, especially if you are involved in writing or research? Well for a start keeping up-to-date goes beyond just reading publications and attending meetings. It is just as important to be able to recall articles quickly, to cite references accurately and to quote from them correctly. To make this easier, you need to do three things:

- acquire the information
- note important information
- store references so they can be easily retrieved.

Acquiring information

Your choice of reading depends of course on your research and general interests. It will cover journals, books, conference and other reports, especially review articles and journals that review papers published within a specialty each month. And do not forget that scanning the index of journals will give you a good idea of published material.

If you need to do a detailed study or review of a subject you should search computerised bibliographic databases such as Medline, about which your librarian will give you advice. *See also* Literature review, p. 66. From such databases you will obtain citations of all your references, and, in many cases, abstracts.

How much time you spend reading new material each week depends on the time you have and the amount of reading you need to do.

Noting important information

This can be done manually with record cards, although most people would now use a computer database. You will need to record:

- the title of the paper
- the authors
- the full title of the journal or book
- the volume number, page numbers and year of publication.
- description of the paper and work (case report or general report, leading article, editorial, review or letter, etc.; results of controlled trial, original study, etc.)
- the institution where the work was carried out
- key words
- an abstract
- the location of material (e.g. your own collection, in the library, etc.).

Much of the above can be done in your particular shorthand or code.

Storing information for retrieval

This is the most difficult of the three tasks but the most important. Your ability to recall the important message from the paper without necessarily reading it all over again will depend on how you file the information.

A database is only an electronic filing cabinet. A database is an organised collection of data on a given subject. The database will be composed of a single data file or several files – a file being a collection of records on a theme. All the records on a given subject make up a file, and all the files together form the database. The record is divided into 'data fields', each holding information on one aspect of the reference, such as the names of the authors, etc., as above. One advantage of the computer database is the ability to search for records on multiple variables, to create index files and to use the system in conjunction with word processing programs. You can either create your own system using the database supplied with your computer software or purchase a separate, more sophisticated package specially designed to handle bibliographic data. These are more expensive but some can communicate with bibliographic databases such as Medline and therefore provide means of obtaining a large number of references from the computer terminal installed in the department or even at home.

Key stages in the writing process

- Developing your idea
- Background reading and literature search
- Conducting the research
- Analysing the results
- Writing

Literature review

One way to review the literature is to work backwards through the journals, either scanning the contents lists for suitable papers or reading some of the review journals. *Index Medicus* can be used for searching for references to a key word or topic. It is published every month and at the end of the year as a *Cumulative Index Medicus.* It has a thesaurus known as MeSH (medical subject headings), which is published in January. This is the key to the whole *Index Medicus*; in effect the index to the index. But it is an American publication so beware of spelling. An alternative is *Excerpta Medica* published in Amsterdam. It too has a thesaurus called *Malimet*.

You may wish to use one of the computerised bibliographic databases, such as Medline, which incorporates all of the constituent journals in *Index Medicus*, or DHSSDATA, which provides Department of Health and Social Security (DHSS) publications. From these you will obtain citations (and in many cases abstracts) of your references. Your first attempt can often be daunting. If you can obtain the help of a qualified librarian then do so. You first need to precisely define your search subject. Are there synonyms? Alternative spellings? You also need to decide how far back you want the search to go. The further back you search, the more you will find and so the more time-consuming it becomes.

Good research needs a framework or a set of stages, not necessarily chronological, which should be systematically addressed whatever the scale of the project. Choosing the topic and formulating the problem that is feasible within the timescale is just one beginning.

Starting the written stages

Aims, objectives or hypotheses

Set out what you want to achieve and how. This will influence your choice of methodological approach and design of the study. The purpose of the research can be set out as a statement of aims or as a research hypothesis, or both. In health research the range of possible methodologies is vast, stretching from classical quantitative or scientific methods through a variety of structured and semi-structured designs and surveys to qualitative approaches. You also need to identify resource implications and may need to seek approval from your local ethical committee.

Pilot study for data collection

Having planned the study, including your forms for data recording, questionnaires, attitude scales, equipment needed to detect flaws in design, etc., a pilot study is essential. When happy with this you can then proceed to full data collection.

Preparation for writing

Having carried out all the work you then need to prepare the data for analysis and present the findings in a structured way. It might be helpful to re-read the section on writing reports (*see* p. 57).

It is also helpful to evaluate and reflect on how the research was carried out and whether parts could have been done differently or better. The research process can be thought of as a cycle, where having worked through all stages you may well find yourself back at the beginning, rethinking the topic and formulation of the study. Each stage is interconnected with every other stage. For example, inadequate funding may mean revision of the scope of the project. To obtain an overview of the process it is helpful to consider each stage independently.

Writing journal articles

Getting yourself published adds greatly to your curriculum vitae. You may also make a contribution to your professional colleagues' understanding. Publishing research results in refereed journals is, obviously, most attractive, but is also difficult. You may learn and grow your confidence by getting an article or two accepted by a non-refereed journal. If you are unsure of how to start, ask more senior colleagues to share their experience with you. Having selected a journal, it is essential to obtain a copy of authors' instructions from the publisher. Study the style and approach of examples of previously successful articles before submitting your own.

Creating structure

Here are ten steps to guide you from initial idea to final article. The actual layout you use will be guided by reference to 'authors' notes' set out by the journal you are aiming at, and also the house style of that journal.

1 Consider all the implications of your idea and ask yourself 'so what am I trying to say?'
2 What do you want a reader to do, say or think after they have read your article? In other words what are you trying to achieve?
3 Make a plan of the points in your argument to ensure the article flows from point to point.
4 Try to capture your reader's interest in the first paragraph.
5 Try to keep your reader's interest by telling them what you are going to say and what you have said.
6 Do not assume others have your level of knowledge, so explain and put them fully in the picture.
7 Discuss, analyse and give reasons for your ideas and arguments.
8 Illustrate by using headings, charts, tables, graphs and pictures, wherever necessary, to clarify and emphasise your points and so break up the text.
9 Summarise and finish by presenting your key conclusions, recommendations and ideas for other readers, prompting further research and discussion.
10 Show a draft to one or more colleagues or friends for comments and honest criticisms then choose the one you want to take notice of because you will inevitably receive contradictory opinions. Maybe also ask advice and help from people who have published before.

Common style issues

• With acronyms, the most common style is to use capitals for each letter pronounced (e.g. BBC and NHSE), otherwise, if pronounced as a single word acronym, use upper and lower case (e.g. Unesco and Aids).
• Capitals slow the reader down and should be kept to a minimum. Avoid pompous initial capitals as in 'the Doctors', 'the Nurses' but 'the patients'. Words like 'Department', 'Authority' and 'Mission Statement' do not need initial capitals.
• Christian names are not appropriate for multiracial societies; it is preferable to use 'first' name.

- Exclamation marks should be used extremely sparingly.
- Avoid stereotyping, for example doctors as male and nurses as female.
- 'Include' is a splendid word for writers because it allows for any complaint that the list is incomplete.
- Monologophobia is the fear of using the same word more than once in the same sentence or passage. This fear is overrated and can lead to confusion when, for example, authors use 'study', 'research' and 'investigation' in one paragraph to describe the same activity.

Some important points to remember.

- Check your spelling and grammar. Nothing spoils credibility more. This is the responsibility of the author, not the typist.
- Avoid padding, which only detracts. Clarity and brevity attract the reader's attention.
- Ensure accuracy.
- Do not make assumptions unless they are clearly stated.
- Check that what you say is justified by evidence from within the report. You may not be there when the reader seeks justification.
- If a sentence requires a lot of punctuation, break it up into shorter sentences.
- Limit yourself to one idea per paragraph.
- Do ask someone else to read it and make comments.

Review

Here are ten questions you could ask yourself about the article after it is written.

1 Is it interesting to read?
2 Is it clearly written?
3 Is it relevant to previous work?
4 Is it built on and relevant to the existing body of knowledge?
5 Is there clear evidence and objectivity?
6 Is there quality and logical progression in your arguments?
7 What are the theoretical and practical implications?
8 Does it meet editorial objectives?
9 Have I left it for a while and then re-read it?
10 Have I asked a few others what they think of it?

When your work has been submitted, what will referees look for in your paper? They will consider all the questions set out above. They will also try to identify both strengths and weaknesses of the methods and examine whether the physical measurements, equipment, questionnaires, attitude scales and so on are appropriate to the question posed. Was there a pilot study and data collection to detect any flaws in the design? With the data preparation and analysis, what analysis was required to test the research hypothesis? Are the data at the appropriate level of measurement for the planned statistical tests? Had it received ethical committee approval? Was the methodology appropriate? Could it have been done differently or better?

It is not just the role of those evaluating research to decide whether or not to make changes or innovations based on the findings. As a practising clinician you need to be able to evaluate papers you read in journals which suggest changes in practice. Researchers make an enormous contribution to innovations and changes in practice, but ultimately they only really provide the mechanism for that consideration.

Action

Do not expect the skills to come easily, particularly at first. Persevere, and learn from your many mistakes – you will find that you have at your disposal an extremely useful tool. Once you are satisfied with a plan, remind yourself of your brief, arm yourself with your plan and start writing. The majority of writers on writing suggest that you write the whole piece (or, if it is a long one, a substantial part of it) in one go. This will ensure that the piece is consistent.

Obtain copies of medico-legal reports carried out by more than one experienced person and study style and layout.

Consider the following and decide whether each is fact, feeling, value or opinion.

- Waiting lists are still too high.
- For the third year, despite our best efforts, waiting lists have increased.
- Waiting lists increased by 5% this year compared with last year.
- Waiting lists have increased substantially.

You may also want to consider writing up a case report of an interesting case or unusual presentation you have seen. You will need to do a literature search to ensure that no one has already written up a whole series.

Or you might consider writing up a useful piece of audit you have been involved in, with a message that deserves wider dissemination..

Next time you read a paper in a journal, consider whether there are any flaws in the work. Was it a valid piece of work, logical, well reasoned, etc.?

Presenting a curriculum vitae

To find the job you want, you need to know and understand the market, which varies among specialties. You can do this by attending meetings, talking to people and doing some investigations. Meanwhile assemble facts for your curriculum vitae (CV). You need to ask yourself the question 'Is it the right job for me?' To do so you need the details, job description and person specification. You might also find it useful to talk to others, including your consultants, who know you, the situation generally, the job and the hospital.

Applications for jobs should be clear and concise, typewritten so that they are easy to read, well prepared and presented, accurate and up to date. They may require submission either via an application form or by a CV, or a mixture of both. The choice for which is used seems to vary. An application form has the advantage of excluding information not relevant to the application, thereby standardising the process and making it fairer and easier for short-listing. CVs leave more scope for the individual to show creativity and initiative. The applicant has more control over the selection process by including information in or excluding information from a CV. Applicants usually prefer CVs. Selectors prefer well-completed standard application forms.

Selection panels generally have time constraints, so help them by being clear and concise and ensuring your CV is typewritten, well prepared, well presented, accurate and up-to-date. It should include personal details, qualifications, specialty experience, general experience, research and publications. Examination results and honours or distinctions, scholarships, prizes and other awards may be listed. It is usual to give a full list of your degrees and other qualifications with dates awarded under this heading. Always add achievements outside your career. Marital status, number of children and nationality are not required on a CV. Items such as General Medical Council (GMC) registration number and whether you have right of abode in the UK could be requested and could therefore be included.

Writing your CV is not a process to be hurried. A word processor makes regularly updating your CV very much easier, and unless you do so it is easy to forget publications or other distinctive experience which will enhance your CV.

It is important to comply with any 'instructions for applicants' sent out by the hospital. Supply the correct number of copies however unreasonable this may seem. Some hospitals require an application form to be completed. This can be a standard form for all members of staff and may therefore seem inadequate for more senior medical posts due to lack of space. It is best to complete the form, referring as necessary to the appropriate page of your CV.

There is debate whether previous appointments should be put in chronological or reverse chronological order. Whatever you decide, include a brief summary of your experience. You may also want to classify these under general and specialty experience. Remember that you may need to emphasise certain parts in the light of the requirements of the job you are applying for.

When recording your publications, accuracy is important. Interviewers occasionally check one or more publications, more for its quality than its existence, and will understandably be unimpressed if they cannot find it. As your publications become more plentiful you may wish to classify them as original papers, abstracts, editorials, chapters in books, books, reviews or letters, etc., and perhaps also note your contribution where there is more than one author. Add posters and presentations at scientific meetings, but only if you delivered the address. Poster displays are often published in abstract form and would thus normally appear under the list of publications, but it is not unreasonable to indicate both under the one heading.

Learned societies and committee membership may include other non-clinical or medical societies if you feel you can justify their inclusion, and committee chairmanship or a period as secretary would indicate managerial experience. Other interests, whether cultural, sporting or recreational, should be mentioned, especially if they feature distinguishing excellence. Team sports give the impression of team membership and a captaincy may suggest team leadership. Similarly, committee membership of a university or hospital club suggests organisational and administrative ability.

A short covering letter should accompany your application, mentioning the post for which you are applying and stating that you are enclosing copies of your CV and the names of referees.

Referees are vital to your application and their choice is therefore important. The choice is likely to be yours, although there is a trend towards requiring your current educational supervisor or supervising consultant to act as one of your referees. The choice requires considerable thought. They obviously need to think highly enough of you to support your application. Referees will sometimes show you the reference they have written for you and this can be very helpful. Ask your referees' permission before submitting your application and supply them with copies of the job description and person specification, plus a copy of your CV. Also supply them with the likely date of the interview, so that if they are away at least their secretary will be able to notify the appointing hospital. It reflects badly on a candidate if the named referee has not sent a reference and it may be assumed that the fault lies with the candidate not having allowed sufficient time.

Presentation skills

Effective communication of ideas is fundamental to the development of professional knowledge. Postgraduate professional development is (in part) dependent on doctors sharing research and knowledge with colleagues in regular meetings. Your ability to make effective presentations can also have a significant effect on your career opportunities, since self-presentation is a key factor in attracting attention to your potential.

For the purpose of this section, presentations are taken to mean any situation in which you are required to communicate information, ideas, propositions or a report to an audience of any size. These might include presenting an audit report to a department, reviewing a paper or contributing to a presentation with others. Making an effective presentation means knowing how to present your ideas, your research and yourself confidently and to the best advantage. Of course, you want to be able to do this without spending too long agonising over it. This section will help you make the most of your opportunities in making a good impression as a presenter in both formal and informal situations. It will do this by taking you through the processes involved in preparing a good presentation. That is, first selecting relevant material, then organising that material and finally delivering it to the best effect.

The first important thing to realise about presentation situations is that, although our basic medium of communication is words, they account for only a small part of the total message. It is generally accepted that less than 25% of what you communicate will be concerned with your words and some 75% will be concerned with the way you use your voice and with body language, such as facial expression, posture and gestures.

You cannot give a good presentation unless you have done the right kind of careful preparation. As part of your preparation you must have the answers to six fundamental questions:

WHY am I speaking?

What is the *purpose* of the talk? Is it to inform, to teach, to make a proposition or to inspire and motivate? Defining your objective, preferably in a single sentence, will make preparation simpler and focus the talk.

To WHOM am I speaking?

The size, mix, level of understanding and attitudes of the audience must be taken into account during preparation. Levels of complexity and volume of information and ideas will depend on the likelihood that members of the audience can absorb them in the time available.

WHERE am I speaking?

Always visit the venue before your presentation unless it is impossible for you to do so. Check the equipment is working, decide where you will stand and whether your voice will carry without a microphone. Remember that the presence of an audience will deaden the impact and volume of your voice. Make sure the seating layout suits the kind of presentation you have in mind.

WHEN am I speaking?

If your presentation is to be made at the end of the working day, you will need to take into account the energy level of members of the audience. The duration of the talk should affect its structure and level of detail. Avoid trying to pack in too much for the audience to absorb in the time available. Audiences will get restless if you run over your allotted time, so keep to your plan. It helps to note the time by which you must finish and to place a watch in front of you at the beginning of your presentation.

WHAT am I going to say?

The content will be determined by the objective. Keep returning to your objective statement in order to avoid losing direction. The material is normally organised in one of the following ways:

- a generalisation followed by detailed explanation/illustration
- using a time, spatial or geographical sequence, or a sequence based on ascending or descending order of importance of each element
- contrasting one set of facts/ideas with another
- dividing a unit up into its component parts and saying a little about each.

Ask yourself which method will help you to present your material most effectively; when you've done that, you are ready to write the first draft. Most good presentations are divided into an introduction, which sets the scene and prepares the audience for what is to come; a main body comprised of three or four main points; and a conclusion, which summarises and emphasises the theme.

- Write your opening and closing sentences in full and learn them 'off by heart'.
- Capture the audience and tell them everything they need to know about the presentation in the opening.
- Make the conclusion really conclusive.

Remember that your presentation will be *spoken*. When you write your draft, write it in spoken English, not written English. This will help you to sound more natural, even when you are actually reading whole phrases or sentences from your cue cards (as most speakers do from time to time).

To help you achieve a clear, natural style remember these tips.

- Use simple, familiar words that come to you naturally.
- Only use technical jargon that your audience will understand.
- Use short sentences.

HOW am I going to say it?

Most speakers use notes or prompt cards, but speak from brief notes to avoid reading word for word. The use of voice and gesture as well as audio-visual aids requires careful thought, practice and self-awareness.

Speaking notes

- Use small cards rather than sheets of paper if possible. They are easier to hold and look more professional.
- Write key sentences and key words on the cards.
- Fasten the cards together, or at least number them in sequence.

Effective delivery

This is achieved by paying attention to articulation, pace, intonation and emphasis.

- Good articulation can be achieved by practising enunciation in front of a mirror. Many speakers are 'lazy' in the way they form their sounds, not moving their lips and tongue enough. Keep your head up. Don't speak with your chin down in your collar.
- Pace should be varied to maintain interest. Nervous speakers always speak too quickly. Avoid racing! Pauses can be used for effect, but they also allow the listeners to absorb the points you are making and react to them.
- Intonation is the rhythm and inflection in the voice. Most people use only two or three tones of the musical scale when they speak. The Welsh and the Western Highlanders, on the other hand, use about an octave and a half. Get colour into your voice.
- Emphasis, often coupled with repetition, is a most useful speaking device. If your voice lacks colour, practise emphasising key words and phrases from your cue cards. Remember that you can also emphasise points by using appropriate (but not distracting) gestures.

In general

- Speak as naturally and conversationally as possible.
- Stand in a comfortable position with your feet slightly apart.
- Smile and be friendly.
- Maintain good eye contact with the whole audience.
- Check whether you have any distracting mannerisms and work to get rid of them. These may include excessive use of certain phrases or sounds such as 'you know', 'Um', 'Er' or 'You see'. Habits such as jingling keys or coins in a pocket, or pacing up and down like a caged tiger, can also be a barrier to effective communication with the audience.

Visual aids

Good use of visual aids will improve your presentation by helping your audience to remember what you have said more easily than if you use words alone. Visual aids used badly or carelessly can be very distracting and even irritating, and are often worse than none at all.

- Check that equipment is in the right place and working properly before you begin.
- Be sure that everything is large enough to be seen by everyone in the room.
- Don't read from visuals – you insult the audience's intelligence.
- Face the audience, not your screen.
- Each picture should have only one main message. Complex slides confuse and bore.
- Minimise the words on each visual. A maximum of 20 is a good rule of thumb.
- Words should be printed and at least 20-point font size should be used.
- Always be prepared with back-up material, to cope if the machinery breaks down.

Handouts are sometimes used to support a presentation. It is generally unhelpful to circulate them at the start of your presentation as they become a distraction.

Taking questions

Decide whether you will take questions during or after your presentation and tell your audience your decision clearly in the introduction to your presentation.

Listen carefully to the question and check that you've understood it. Repetition of the question also helps everyone in the room to know exactly what is being answered. Do not expect questions to come as soon as you stop talking. You are expecting the audience to go into a different mode, so be prepared to wait or 'plant' a question in the audience to get things going. Keep your answers short as you may bore the rest of the audience.

Exercise

Bearing in mind the above notes, describe in the space below what you see as your strengths and weaknesses as a presenter. If possible seek pointers from a colleague or friend who has seen you make presentations.

Strengths:

Weaknesses:

Now reflect on these, considering which of your weaknesses could be due to lack of experience or learning, and which are unchangeable. Seek to describe them in ways which help you to decide what improvements you need to make in your approach.

Now identify the types of situation in which you expect to make presentations over the next year or so:

At your next presentation, ask a couple of members of the audience (preferably friends who you can rely on to give you helpful feedback) to make notes about the way you make your presentation and tell you what they thought of it afterwards. You and they may find the checklist (below) useful as a guide. Do not mention your perceived weaknesses to them beforehand, but quiz them about these aspects of your presentation when you get your feedback.

Good luck!

Presentation Feedback Sheet

Content

- Introduction
  - was the purpose clear?
  - was a link made with the audience?
  - did the speaker make an impact within the first two minutes?

- Main body
  - was the talk pitched at a level to suit the audience?
  - were there clear stages?
  - did it follow a logical sequence?

- Conclusions
  - was there a summary of key points?
  - (if relevant) was there an indication of action to be taken, and by whom?

Voice

- Volume too loud/soft?
- Tone varied to maintain interest?
- Pace too fast/slow?

Timing

- Start and finish on time?

Stance

- Relaxed posture, facing audience.

Mannerisms

- Free from distraction, such as pacing, verbal habits, etc.

Visual aids

- Relevant/simple and clear/technically proficient?

Contributing to meetings

Meetings are a feature of professional life. They are a common event for clinicians representing colleagues, nurse managers and business managers. They are also expensive. They can waste time, for example when there is no clear objective to the meeting, or a lack of effective leadership and control, or there are too many or the wrong participants. Time is often wasted on debate about 'Why?' rather than 'How?'. In addition, a lack of clarity on outcomes produces unclear final decisions or even no decisions. Meetings which do not achieve results not only waste time, but can even lead to more meetings.

Types of meeting

There are many different kinds of meeting, including small group, support, events, clinical, staff, departmental, open or public, committees, workshops, learning sessions, conferences and so on. Every well-run meeting, whether formal or informal, is based on three pre-requisites:

- clear aims
- careful planning
- effective teamwork.

Aims

Clear aims will be related to the purpose of the meeting. A departmental meeting may be for talking, listening and sharing problems. A committee normally aims to make and agree decisions, whereas a learning session is about sharing ideas through teaching and learning.

Always go to meetings knowing what you want to achieve. Advance preparation is vital and that applies to all participants. How often have you been at a presentation of a new idea and when participants have been asked to comment, nearly everyone has suggestions for improvements? No one had been given the opportunity to study the proposal in advance, everyone was seeing it for the first time. Discussions are lengthy and suggestions numerous. Other time wasters include fighting losing or lost battles by discussing items decided elsewhere or that are not within the group's power to decide.

Some reasons for meetings

Meetings can be called for all sorts of reasons other than reaching a decision, and these can be classified as follows:

- creating and developing ideas, for example brainstorming sessions
- sharing out work and responsibility, usually valuable for small groups only
- delegation of work or authority within a group
- sharing responsibility for a difficult problem
- providing or receiving information – there may be better ways
- persuasion – best done before the meeting

- networking, which become 'talking shops'
- an alternative to preparing a short written report
- committees in the habit of meeting without a real purpose, even with lengthy agendas
- socialising – acceptable at the beginning of a meeting, but do keep it short
- perhaps as a substitute for work.

Decision making at meetings

Decision making on tasks or issues may be a valid reason for calling a meeting, but you need to ask yourself if it is:

- consulting before a decision is made
- gathering information for a decision to be made elsewhere
- gaining agreement on a decision
- seeking a decision that requires the agreement of more than one group
- enhancing commitment to a decision
- making a decision.

Why go to a meeting?

Any meeting you attend is your meeting too. Do you know why you're going? At every meeting you should have a personal objective(s).

Planning for a meeting

Make sure you are fully prepared otherwise you are failing to be an effective member. It may be the opportunity to put across a message. A seed sown today might be important for later. You can often turn someone else's question into a bridge for your own message. A question directed at you, in any situation, will always give you an opportunity to say what you want. Always answer the question and then make your point. If you are asked a question and you don't know the answer it is perfectly acceptable to say: 'I don't know but I'll find out and let you know' and then go on to your statement, via a suitable link. You can also use the same technique in response to a statement, by agreeing with that statement, before linking to your own statement. Here the speaker becomes the leader and controls the meeting while speaking. This is observable at medical committees.

Seating arrangements

Semicircles are good for problem-solving meetings and provide a good balance of control and sensitivity for the leader. Long tables are control mechanisms and inhibit brainstorming sessions. It is impossible to see others down the same side of the table and discussions between participants is limited. The more eye contact and with more people, the more control you have. To some extent where you sit will depend on your purpose. If you want to be uninvolved pick a position that permits that. If you are seeking to win a point or plan seizing control, pick a controlling position. At a long table this will be at either end. At a three-sided arrangement this will be either side of the chair or at either end. At a long table, an ally at the other end of the table will give you maximum support in handling a difficult meeting. Next time you are at a meeting observe where people sit and see how it influences their roles. If you are going to be a competitor to the chair, sit as far away as possible. The ideal position is opposite so that you can talk directly to the chair and include others as well.

General meeting techniques

Interruptions

Knowing when to interrupt to gain control is a useful tool.

- 'Could I add ...' and continue speaking.
- Call the person by name, 'John, don't forget ...', and continue speaking.
- Just start speaking and raise your voice above the level of the other person.

Do not wait for permission to be granted before you interrupt, but continue talking. It is often difficult to hang back while someone presents something which you consider inappropriate. But do think twice before making yourself vulnerable by interrupting the speaker, as your own point may not be quite as perfect as you thought.

If you want to prevent yourself being interrupted:

- insist on finishing by saying: 'Please, just let me finish ...' and continue
- hold your hand up, palm outwards, and continue.

Criticism

If you should be the subject of criticism, ask the critic to present an analysis of your proposal with workable alternatives for the next meeting. Emotion can resist logic. When someone is emotionally aroused, your best ploy is to remain silent until their emotion peters out.

Opposition

When you are up against opposition your objective should always be to determine your opponent's objectives. There is nothing wrong with having a different objective. Ask yourself what your opponent wants and why they want it. Only then can you plan your own strategy.

Confrontation

If you are disagreeing with someone try to provide your opponent with a way out, a way to save face. If you disagree, first state what you agree with, thus supporting their position as modified by your own. Make criticism less personal by claiming you are acting as the 'devil's advocate'.

Contribute early

Research has indicated that when a person contributes early in a discussion, they are more likely to exert a greater influence throughout the discussion. This forces opponents to respond to you, but be prepared to come back into the discussion to combat opposing points when you rebut their counter arguments.

Defending a weak case

Sometimes you may find yourself defending a case which you believe to be right but for which you have little evidence as yet. When your case is weak, consider additional techniques such as psychology of the seating. Associate your opposer's idea with a word or phrase that has negative connotations. Use glittering generalities that associate positive images with your idea. Use transference where you buttress your idea by reference to respected authorities. Use audio-visual aids to divert attention away from the substance of your idea. The group may vote on the presentation rather than the substance.

When you are winning, do not waste everyone's time by continuing the argument.

Action

There is an important difference between a stimulating discussion and a productive meeting. For the next meeting you attend, ask yourself:

- what is the purpose of this meeting?
- what should I achieve by the end?
- how will I distinguish my success from failure?

After the meeting ask yourself:
- was I correct about the task?
- were the other participants clear about the task and objectives?
- did I achieve the meeting's objective as stated in the agenda?
- was the meeting a success or failure?
- if not, why not?
- what could be done to improve the next meeting?
- what was done that should be discontinued?
- what could the chairperson do to improve the meeting?
- could you have done without the meeting?
- if so, how?

Being interviewed

Prepare everything the day before and allow plenty of time by arriving early and having all possible questions and your answers totally revised and memorised. You need to convince the panel that you will achieve your goals or, in the cases of a consultant appointment, make a delightful colleague.

The size of appointment committees tends to grow, although there are guidelines and statutory regulations for the composition of selection committees. Apart from consultants within a specialty, members of the selection committee will not all know one another. So you can be reassured that even some of the panel members may feel in strange surroundings. And many panel members confess privately to nervousness too!

As a general rule you should dress to reassure and fit the stereotype of the post for which you have applied. Go into the room positively, smiling and determined to enjoy it. It will not be as bad as a viva examination. Try to:

- be relaxed but business-like
- sit upright
- be friendly, smile with perhaps a degree of authority
- look initially at the chair, who should put you at your ease
- show enthusiasm for the job.

Interview questions

Routine questions (usually from the chair) about your journey or finding the place help to 'break the ice' and are usually followed by some more routine questions to clarify any queries with your CV, such as unusual features or gaps. The questions then tend to move on to asking you your reasons for wanting the job or what attracted you to it. This is an opportunity to show that you have researched the hospital. Have you identified any challenge that the institution faces? This leads naturally to where you see your career going or how you see it developing. Be enthusiastic and do not give evasive answers. The questions are invariably not difficult, but simply attempting to get you to talk about yourself. Do so with a mixture of:

- confidence
- intelligence
- charm
- humour
- enthusiasm
- honesty
- maturity

as appropriate to the question. Address your answer initially to the questioner but look around and try to engage all the panel with your answer.

Be neither monosyllabic nor loquacious; balance is important. Even if asked closed questions avoid the temptation to give simple 'yes' or 'no' answers. Try and expand the answer to allow the interviewer time to recover You will gain no friends by making him or her feel uncomfortable.

The panel will normally have agreed in advance to split up questions into a number of areas, each covered by one panel member. You might be asked about your vision of the hospital and department, what you think of the hospital or what have you to offer. Typical questions ask about research you have done or intend to do, your experience of clinical audit, government reports which affect you and the NHS generally, as well as possible future plans and changes in NHS.

There may be questions that reveal 'what makes the candidate tick'. These are usually about hobbies and outside interests. Avoid suggesting these might interfere with your work! Aptitudes and outside interests are a measure of whether you are a well-rounded personality.

Talking about strengths and weaknesses

They may try to reveal your virtues and weaknesses, perhaps by asking about your mistakes or weakness directly, or your aptitudes and ambitions. Answers tend to reveal your personal values. Questions about weakness, mistakes, tasks that you could have done better or opportunities missed gauge your self-awareness, intellectual honesty, maturity and dependability, and may relate indirectly to your team-membership characteristics. There are no right answers to these questions. But it is worth thinking in advance about mistakes you have made, difficult situations you have been in and times when you have felt out of your depth and hope you coped, and what you learned from these experiences. Pressure questions about previous failed interviews may also give clues about your ability to cope with stress, your maturity and your emotional stability.

Questions about your greatest achievements, challenges or responsibilities are an attempt to obtain a record of your standards, your qualities of management and relationships, as well as your leadership style and ability, and whether you are a process- or people-oriented person. Questions about relationships are trying to assess relationships with colleagues by view of personality: social or self-contained; conforming or independent; extrovert or sensitive; phlegmatic or excitable.

Handling difficult panel members

They are the ones who ask tricky questions that are intended to impress the committee with the questioner's skill. If you are asked that sort of question, stay calm and if you find you are struggling remember that only better candidates get asked difficult questions to separate them, and that committee members usually have sympathy for candidates being given a difficult time by colleagues.

Handling silence

If there is silence after your answer you are being invited to continue. Do not be embarrassed by silence, even if you need time to think about your answer. Allow yourself time to think before answering so that your replies are considered and logical. Do not be tempted to leap in and say something ill-considered. You need not be embarrassed to have a question clarified if you are not clear what you are being asked, but do not waste time looking for hidden catches. Remember the interviewers are usually seeking reassurance. Do make sure you are answering the question asked. With multiple questions try to remember the individual questions or clarify before answering.

Conclusion

Try to appear friendly, cheerful and smiling. Body language helps with a business-like authoritative attitude, professional appearance and energetic approach. At the end of the interview you are generally invited by the chair to ask the panel any questions you might have. While it will not count against you to ask a question, it is acceptable and possibly desirable not to do so.

Panel presentations

This is a developing method of helping to assess candidates for consultant appointments and is thought to be a reasonable way of assessing the vision of candidates in relation to the future of a unit. Whether the candidate has grasped the problems of the unit in pre-interview visits and has a realistic expectation of what they are coming to will also be apparent. Some candidates like it as a way of being in control of the first half of the interview, whereas others feel uncomfortable making presentations, particularly as it will not usually be a part of their everyday work. It does illustrate the importance of making sure you collect useful information from the clinical director, medical director, chief executive and chairman when paying your pre-application visit.

Information in the NHS

This section will help you to understand the role of information in the NHS and the use of information technology in teaching and training, clinical decision making and research.

Exciting advances in new technologies are continuously being introduced. Telemedicine and diagnostic computer systems are challenging the need for some conventional hospital facilities. Computerised decision support systems designed to aid decision making have not always lived up to expectations. Such systems function as sophisticated information tools for clinicians rather than replacing clinical decision makers.

Computers can be used to support team working and ensure continuity of care, for example by making the complete past medical history of a patient readily available. Problems of privacy, breaches of data confidentiality and lack of integration due to the multiplicity of systems have delayed progress. Separate systems exist for primary care, biochemistry, haematology, radiology and imaging and administration.

The NHS is a very large, complex organisation comprising a great number of smaller organisations which operate (frequently independently of each other) to plan, fund and provide healthcare. Efficient provision of effective care requires close collaboration and good communication at all levels. This requires a flow of information that is accurate, up-to-date and relevant, together with an agreed interpretation of its meaning. Information combined with interpretation represents knowledge and the NHS employs the knowledge to provide healthcare for patients. The management of knowledge is of fundamental importance to all aspects of the NHS.

Doctors are increasingly expected to provide expert guidance to patients who, after browsing the Internet, may be better informed about their condition than their doctor. For many doctors this requires a radical rethink of attitudes. Searching through medical research journals may be replaced by accessing large electronic databases published on the Internet. This brings into question the relative roles of doctors and other related professionals. The management of knowledge is, perhaps, one of the most challenging aspects of the new technologies.

As patterns of clinical practice continue to change in the light of the new technology (for example, increased use of day surgery units, one-stop clinics, multi-specialty community care) the information needs of the NHS also change. It is important that everyone in the NHS has sufficient familiarity with information technology (IT) to enable them to work effectively and efficiently, and it is equally important that existing IT systems are developed to meet the future needs of the NHS. This will only happen if future users are involved in creating the systems that meet their needs.

In 1998, the NHSE launched an information strategy for the NHS. It was seen as a key enabler to reforms in the NHS. It encouraged, for example, support telephone-based services such as NHS Direct and online services which would allow GPs to book hospital appointments and access test results more easily.

In 1998, around 85% of GP practices were computerised. Development of clinical systems had occurred in a sizeable minority of acute hospitals, in addition to the development of a national infrastructure to support the:

- NHS patient number – to identify individual patients
- NHSnet – the NHS's own network on the Internet
- NHS-wide clearing service – dealing with service agreements.

A special health authority, known as the NHS Information Authority, was set up in 1999 to take over responsibility from the Information Management Group for the issue of IT in the NHS.

Use of IT in the NHS

Information technology is used in the NHS in broadly three ways:

- administration
- research and training
- diagnosis.

Computer-based (digital) information systems have been available for around 30 years and have found uses in virtually every corner of the NHS.

One advantage of using digital information is that it can be transmitted electronically from one computer to another. Two or more computers connected together in this way is called a network. A computer can be linked into a network directly using a specific hardware interface, or indirectly using a conventional telephone line. However, passing information through a telephone connection is usually much slower because digital information has to be translated into sound before it can be sent along the telephone cables. Using a network reduces duplication of equipment and information and allows faster communication of up-to-date information. Networks can serve just a local area (LAN) or they can be truly global (e.g. Internet, World Wide Web).

The NHS national network – NHSnet

This is a secure national network developed exclusively for the NHS. It consists of a national core network provided by BT with regional networks supplied by BT and Cable & Wireless. As well as carrying communications between all parts of the NHS it supports a number of services:

- NHS message handling
- NHS-wide clearing
- secure, high-speed Internet access
- national e-mail system with electronic address books.

There has been reluctance to connect from some NHS organisations because of concerns about cost.

Privacy, security and confidentiality

Wider adoption of IT in the NHS has also possibly been held back by concerns over privacy, security and confidentiality of personal health data. The Caldicott Committee (1997) published a report suggesting that more patient identifiable information was transmitted than necessary. It also suggested nomination of a senior member of staff as 'Caldicott guardian', to protect patient confidentiality and prevent unnecessary identification of patients. The Caldicott implementation steering group oversees the implementation of these matters in addition to seeking technical solutions on security.

National Framework for Assessing Performance (NFAP)

This framework for assessing performance is a new way of evaluating the service in six areas:

- health improvement
- fair access
- effective delivery of appropriate healthcare
- efficiency
- patient/carer experience
- health outcomes.

The NHS is developing new indicators and data sets to add to existing performance measures, as well as creating processes to ensure that indicators can be generated from operational systems supporting clinical care. This involves finding ways of collecting patient data which is consistent and comparable in a common language for clinicians and managers.

Read codes and clinical data standards

Common record structures, terminology and protocols for the capture and communication of clinical information are necessary to develop patient-based records compatible with information systems. A clinical information management programme (CIMP) will attempt to build on existing work out of developing Read codes. The suitability of the codes is being assessed and it seems likely that, by 2002, the use of Read codes in clinical systems will become mandatory.

IT systems and NHS administration

Systems in use for the administration of patient care can be separated into two broad types: patient administration systems (PAS) and clinical information systems (CIS). Access to such systems is usually provided through terminals placed in restricted areas and protected by security procedures, e.g. user accounts and passwords.

Patient administration systems (PAS)

These systems are used in primary and secondary healthcare organisations and at the basic level hold a list of patients' demographic details. Within a hospital, the PAS is used to link the patient demographics with the hospital case note number, and usually also used to manage outpatient appointments, waiting lists and other purely administrative tasks.

Clinical information systems (CIS)

There is a wide range of electronic information systems that manage clinical information. The functions of such systems have been classified into resource management (RM), quality and audit (QA), clinical management support (CMS), and electronic patient records (EPR). Clinical systems may be hospital-wide (for example, hospital information system (HIS)) or implemented at a departmental level (for example, radiology information system (RIS)).

The primary roles of these systems are to record and analyse the clinical workload of the hospital, to provide information for the management of the NHS at both local and national levels, and to compare actual with planned performance. Resource management systems control the quantity of services provided, audit systems and monitor their quality. The effectiveness of both systems is critically dependent on the accuracy and completeness of the information entered for each patient. Information collection for resource management and quality assurance must be integrated into the clinical management process and should avoid excessive paperwork and duplication of effort.

Clinical management support (CMS) and electronic patient records (EPR)

Clinical management support systems provide access to information used in the diagnosis and treatment of patients. Direct access to the results of diagnostic tests is the most common use and information links to different departments (e.g. pathology, radiology) are usually integrated into a hospital information system. CMS systems may also include the ability to request tests, prescribe drugs and record clinical measurements.

Systems that completely replace the physical records with an electronic patient record (EPR) have considerable potential. To date, only sub-components of such systems have been adopted. One such example is the use of radiology picture archive and communication systems (PACS). The government has stated that it is to invest heavily in the use of IT in the NHS, and a primary objective is that by 2005 all acute hospitals will have established EPR systems.

Electronic technology in teaching, training, clinical practice and research

The use of IT in clinical teaching, training, decision making and research is relatively new, in contrast to its use in administration.

IT in training

The trend has been towards a shorter period of more structured postgraduate education, using distance learning supported by task-oriented training courses. Computer-assisted learning (CAL) has a lot to offer this style of training and the cost of designing good quality CAL programs has become less prohibitive. Some textbooks are now available in digital CD-ROM format. Computer networks can provide shared access to remote sources of interactive, multimedia clinical teaching material that can be developed and kept up-to-date by a team of experienced clinical teachers. The development of such systems requires clinical teachers to be formally trained to make the best use of existing and future IT.

There is increased use of electronic training records, e.g. surgical logbooks, which allows local, regional and national analysis of the quantity and quality of clinical experience available for training. Just as with clinical practice, it is only through collection and sharing of information that improvements can be planned, agreed and implemented.

IT in clinical decision making

Doctors need to work comfortably with and understand computer technology. Once science enables us to know our own genome, we will be able to anticipate future health problems, adapt behaviour to minimise risk, and have treatments personalised. The potential of genetic testing techniques and manipulation of genes is likely to transform the framework that underpins the current clinical medical practice of diagnosis and treatment to prediction and prevention. Gene therapy offers another possible approach. These developments are not without problems, particularly ethical ones such as the destruction of embryos with disabling disorders. The proliferation of genetic testing may also fuel genetic discrimination at work and in financial services such as life insurance. The complexities of biological interactions between genes may, however, make this a more distant prospect than first suggested by pundits.

As always, there is the question of whether the presumed benefits of these new technologies will outweigh the costs. New devices and treatments may cause unanticipated harm and the future of many new technologies remains uncertain. Diseases frequently have multiple causes, and decisions about treatment may involve significant risk analysis. Some decisions, once thought to be easier through using IT and computer science, may become more, rather than less, challenging.

IT and clinical data access

The National Electronic Library of Health (NeLH) aims to provide every professional in the NHS with online access via NHSnet to data on current clinical practice, evidence-based clinical information and help and support with continuing professional development.

Initially, regional libraries were intended to lead the way with a combination of funding from the public and private sectors. One of the main sources of data is The National Institute for Clinical Excellence (NICE). The aim is for the library to carry the full electronic text of the main medical journals and established healthcare databases. Accredited health information and 'virtual' libraries are also being developed for public access.

IT in research

The primary objectives of NHS-based research are to provide clinicians with the skills of critical appraisal and project management, and to update the shared body of knowledge and improve clinical care.

IT has a lot to offer the clinical researcher and when used effectively can greatly increase the efficiency of the time devoted to research. The applications that are of most use are listed in Table 3.1 and Table 3.2 lists when they are used.

Table 3.1 Commonly used IT tools in clinical research

Word processor (WP)	A writing tool that produces high-quality printed documents which can be typed and modified quickly and can include pictures and charts as well as text
E-mail (EM)	For writing and sending electronic messages quickly using a computer linked to a network or modem without printing onto paper. Messages can be copied and circulated to other users and documents, charts and pictures can be sent with the message
Database (DB)	Provides the functions of a card index system but with many additional features. Useful for holding a set of addresses or references
Spreadsheet (SS)	Used to organise, process and present numerical data. Useful for statistical analysis and creating graphs
Presentation generator (PG)	Allows the creation of visual materials and slides for use during presentations. Can be used with a computer projector to give electronic presentations (e.g. Microsoft PowerPoint)
Project management (PM)	An electronic time and resource management application. Useful for large projects where careful co-ordination is important

Table 3.2 Uses of IT tools in the different phases of clinical research

Planning	Remote access to databases of existing publications, e.g. Medline (EM) Fast communication via e-mail (EM) Personal set of published references (DB) Writing project proposal, ethical committee and grant applications (WP)
Execution	Project/time/resource management (PM) Data recording (WP, SS, DB) Data analysis (DB, SS) Data presentation, e.g. graphs or charts (SS, PG) Interim reports, presentations and discussion (WP, SS, PG)
Delivery	Dissertation/thesis (WP, SS, PG) Oral slide presentations (PG) Publications: letters, papers, articles, chapters, books (WP) Teaching materials (WP, PG)

Telemedicine and NHS Direct

Telemedicine allows patients to receive treatment or professionals to seek advice from specialists over long distances using standard telephone technology. The benefits are already proven in the USA where larger distances are involved, but it is still at a relatively early stage of development in the UK.

NHS Direct is a telephone-based help-line for members of the public who have a potential emergency or health enquiry. The staff, who are healthcare professionals, are supported by online databases and links to health services and other specialist helplines.

Information for patients: The Centre for Health Information Quality (CHiQ)

Started in 1997 and originally funded for three years by the NHSE, CHiQ aims to improve high-quality information about services, treatment options and medical outcomes for patients, patients' representatives and self-help organisations. The website address is www.centreforhiq.demon.co.uk.

Developing IT skills

Developing the necessary skills to make best personal use of IT requires more of an investment in time than in equipment, and the earlier the investment is made the greater the potential benefit. Ideally you will have a real need to use IT, such as a research project. This is likely to provide the necessary motivation to complete the learning and integrate it into practice. Essential components are a period of structured training, access to technology and a clear goal to attain relevant IT skills as part of the project. A combination of books, local courses and direct supervision allow you to focus on skills which are most useful to your project. Progression from simpler tasks (e.g. e-mail, word processing and slide presentations) towards the more complex (e.g. spread sheets, databases and project management) provides positive feedback and avoids frustration.

Exercise

Consider what your information requirements would be if you wanted to monitor the performance of your own service.

- List where the information would come from, how it is stored and transmitted, where it goes and for what purpose it is used.
- Identify the points where information is duplicated, lost or distorted.
- Assign priorities for improving the quality of the information management.

Consider how you could use sources of information to improve your own knowledge and the knowledge of the teams in which you work.

- List the most useful sources of information and assess how accessible they are.
- List your current use of information for training and education purposes.
- Identify opportunities for using existing sources of information to improve knowledge.
- Identify sources of likely support for you to develop your own IT skills.

Related reading

Albert T (1996) Effective writing. In: A White (ed) *Textbook of Management for Doctors*. Churchill Livingstone, London. A lot of useful tips on style and grammar.

Albert T (2000) *Winning the Publications Game: how to get published without neglecting your patients* (2e). Radcliffe Medical Press, Oxford.

Allison GT (1971) *Essence of Decision. Explaining the Cuban Missile Crisis*. Little, Brown and Company, Boston. A fascinating insight into meetings at the very highest level and well worth reading in its own right.

BMA (1994) *Guidelines for Good Practice in the Recruitment & Selection of Doctors*. BMA, London.

Buzan T (1989) *Use Your Head*. BBC Books, London.

DoH (1994) *Managing the New NHS: functions and responsibilities*. DoH, London.

DoH (1994) *Research and Development in the New NHS*. DoH, London.

DoH (1996) *Promoting Clinical Effectiveness*. DoH, London.

EL(95) *Priorities and Planning Guidance for the NHS, 1996/7*.

Gatrell J and White T (2000) *Medical Appraisal, Selection and Revalidation*. Royal Society of Medicine, London.

Greenhalgh T (1997) There is a useful series of 11 articles in the *BMJ* beginning **315**: 80.

Gulleford J (1994) Preparing medical experts for the courtroom. No need to learn by trial and error. *BMJ*. **309**: 752–3.

Gowers E (1986) *The Complete Plain Words* (3e). Revised by S Greenbaum and J Whitcut. HMSO, London.

Harris D, Peyton R and Walker M (1996). Teaching in different situations. In: *Training the Trainers: learning and teaching*. Royal College of Surgeons, London.

Klauser HA (1987) *Writing on Both Sides of the Brain*. Harper Collins, San Francisco, CA.

Roberts REI (1994) The trials of an expert witness. *Journal of Royal Society of Medicine*. **87**: 628–31.

White A and Gatrell J (1996) Being interviewed. In: A White (ed) *Textbook of Management for Doctors*. Churchill Livingstone, London.

White A (1996) Managing meetings. In: A White (ed) *Textbook of Management for Doctors*. Churchill Livingstone, London.

4

Non-clinical involvement

with patients

The aim of this chapter is to guide you through the process of obtaining consent, breaking bad news, handling patient complaints and dealing with administrative aspects of post-mortems and coroners' inquests.

Consent

Consent means more than simply getting a signature on the consent form. The patient should be given sufficient information to understand the procedure and be fully aware of what can go wrong. Sometimes this will not be possible due to the condition of the patient immediately before the procedure is to be carried out.

Issues to consider are:

- was the consent fully informed?
- was the patient competent to give consent?
- was consent voluntarily given?

Informed consent

To obtain informed consent, doctors need to explain procedures in detail to patients. A situation frequently faced by juniors is the task of telling a patient what the procedure is, what problems there might be and what can be done about those problems. In this situation theoretical knowledge cannot replace practical experience. Dealing with patients in obtaining consent provides an important learning opportunity.

If the basic requirements have not been met and something goes wrong, the door is open for litigation and the recent growth in litigation is something of which all doctors are aware. These days people are more likely to demand information about their operations and more likely to sue if things go wrong or they feel they had not been given enough information. Doctors need to warn patients of the risks, and it is prudent to advise them with more information than perhaps a court would demand. Ideally, the surgeon carrying out the procedure should be the one to obtain consent. This should ensure that the patient receives all the information they need. There is also the need to remember that patients may be extremely nervous or unable to understand fully the implications of what they are being told.

Many problems may be avoided by obtaining consent when listing patients for elective surgery. Many consultants discuss the procedure with the patient at this time, so it makes sense to obtain consent at the same time, although sometimes it is not clear exactly what patients will need before they come into hospital. There is also a problem if a long period of waiting ensues before admission.

Certainly for more major or complex procedures, consent should be obtained by someone more senior, if only because there can be more complications. If you do not understand the operation, then obtain consent by asking someone more senior who does understand. You should use every opportunity possible to develop your skill in dealing with patients at this stage. Ask to sit in with experienced consultants when they have to obtain consent in difficult circumstances.

Emergencies and absence of consent

A doctor can, in certain circumstances, be justified in providing treatment without consent. The legal ground on which this is based is that of necessity; where consent is 'implied' or 'presumed' or can be assumed to be obtained in the future. Thus a life-saving procedure may be performed where a patient cannot provide consent and is not known to object to the performance of that procedure. As a general rule, treatment given to a patient without consent should be the minimum amount necessary, and any treatment which could reasonably be postponed should be delayed.

In extreme circumstances, common law precedent has enabled doctors to proceed without a patient's consent but the precise scope of that protection is unclear. Medico-legal guidelines indicate that actions of battery, in respect of surgical or other medical treatment, are likely to be confined to cases where surgery or treatment has been performed or given with no consent at all, or where (emergency situations aside) surgery or treatment has been performed or given beyond that to which there is consent.

Permanently incompetent patients

A court is unlikely to deny the right of an incompetent patient to the same appropriate treatment competent patients can expect to receive. The guidelines suggest the following.

- Proceed only if there is agreement on the need for treatment.
- The consent of the nearest relative may be sought, although this has no validity in law.
- If the treatment is for mental disorder, the patient should be treated as if 'temporarily incompetent'.
- Treatment should be administered only if urgently necessary.

Consent for medical research

Generally you will need to be advised by, and seek the formal and written approval of, your hospital's ethical committee in order to carry out such patient research.

This is a matter of some ethical debate and we refer you to articles written in the *BMJ* for 28 March 1998, **316**: 1000–11. These were included as a result of an invitation to comment on this subject a year earlier, which resulted in the generation of considerable correspondence. It covers various views of informed consent in this context, as well as dealing with a publisher's duty and the question of photographs and videos. There are articles by doctors, researchers and medical ethicists, as well as those who represent the views of patients and potential patients.

Consent for photographs and videos

The BMA, the GMC and the Institute of Medical Illustrators all publish guidelines indicating that patients have the right to be given as much information as possible on where an image might be used. Their consent should be obtained prior to all medical photography as well as for subsequent use in a publication, whether they can be identified or not. Specific consent should also be obtained if the image is to be used in electronic publishing. A patient consent form is available on the website www.bmj.com.

Medical negligence

Legal actions in negligence arise when a person who owes a duty of care to another person, because of their relationship (e.g. a doctor and patient), breaches that duty and causes loss or suffering to occur as a result of the breach. Hospital trusts are vicariously liable for employees' actions carried out in the course of their employment. Doctors are therefore not normally sued directly. Medical defence organisations have no role in litigation against NHS hospitals because from 1990, NHS hospitals began indemnifying their employees against patients' allegations of medical negligence. Trusts thus became defendants in legal proceedings and the NHS accepted financial responsibility for claims. When a patient issues proceedings, the health authority or trust – depending on the date of treatment – is the named defendant.

NHS indemnity provides invaluable support to doctors facing litigation. It is, however, strictly limited in its scope. These limits apply not only to civil litigation. It does not indemnify doctors in respect of disciplinary proceedings within the NHS or brought by the GMC. In the former instance, the relevant NHS body is likely to use its own lawyers to prepare a disciplinary case against a doctor. Criminal proceedings are occasionally undertaken against doctors. The NHS provides no indemnity in such cases, but defence bodies, at their discretion, may be prepared to fund such representation. Doctors providing any private treatment, whether in an NHS hospital or elsewhere, will become a named defendant because they have a legal relationship with the patient separate from NHS indemnity.

Although NHS indemnity covers you for the consequences of alleged negligence in NHS hospital or community work in the UK, you could be at risk from the following:

- claims arising out of Category 2 work, including insurance medical reports, medico-legal reports and signing cremation certificates
- disciplinary procedures by your trust or the GMC
- 'Good Samaritan' acts outside the hospital
- lack of access to 24–hour ethical and medico-legal advice line
- criminal charges as a result of your practice within the NHS.

So it is prudent for doctors to maintain their own indemnity to cover those instances where their employer's indemnity may not help, or where the employer may even act against them.

The potential size of the problem

The number of clinical negligence claims against the NHS has grown enormously. In summarised accounts for the NHS in England in 1996/7, £235m was paid out for clinical negligence by health authorities and trusts, and a further £65m paid out by the Department of Health. In a report on the NHS summarised accounts for 1996/7 in 1998, the comptroller and auditor general estimated that the total potential liability of the NHS and the Department for clinical negligence could reach £2.3bn as at March 1997. In addition, the growing cost of legal aid for patients has grown. In 1992/3, it stood at £20m. By 1995/6, it was around £50m.

The NHS Litigation Authority

This special health authority was set up in 1995 to oversee the Clinical Negligence Scheme for Trusts (CNST), a voluntary pooling scheme to assist trusts in managing their clinical negligence liabilities from then on. Most claims for clinical negligence are not well founded and by one reckoning (Evans 1999) only two-fifths of clinical negligence cases finalised in 1996/7 resulted in damages being paid.

Action for Victims of Medical Accidents (AVMA)

AVMA was started in 1982 to provide independent advice and support to patients injured and harmed during the course of medical treatment. It is estimated that in the region of 320 000 adverse events occur each year in hospitals within England, with 40 000 deaths and 20 000 cases of serious disability (Vincent 1995).

Breaking bad news

It is an unfortunate consequence of working in healthcare that you will be called on to be the bearer of upsetting information from time to time. Breaking bad news requires expertise, knowledge, skill and also compassion. You should give careful thought to your own perspective on the kinds of issues that will arise for the person receiving the bad news.

The basic principles

Who

The consultant is normally the lead person but does not necessarily need to be the person who does it. Make sure you are clear about what the person is to be told. Remember the recipient may like to have another person with them. This could be a relative or friend, or someone for support, such as priest or social worker.

Where

Ideally a specially designated area should be used. In any event, it must be private. An office might suffice but ensure there are no interruptions from people entering, the telephone ringing or from your bleep. Try to arrange for comfortable seating without the barrier of a desk.

How

Give information at the earliest appropriate opportunity. Lead in with 'What have you been told already?', 'I've come to discuss your situation', 'Do you know what I have come for?' or 'What have they told you already?' Avoid medical jargon. Patients and families will be confused so don't make it even worse. Be honest, if you do not know something, say so. But let them know if there is someone who does. Check their understanding and when you have finished, make sure there is someone to accompany them after your meeting.

Use appropriate eye contact, voice tone and body language. Ensure that you know what the recipient wants to know and that the time is appropriate for them. Make sure that all people being told are given the same information, with the same options, including an offer of a second opinion. The information should be factual. Do not use 'off-the-cuff' remarks. Give recipients an opportunity to return for further information or clarification.

Ensure that time is allocated not just to breaking the news but to supporting the recipient. In order to ensure that the patient's GP can deal effectively with them, make sure he or she is informed promptly of what the patient has been told. Your hospital will have a timescale for this, normally within two days. The medical record should be fully updated with notes of your consultation with the patient.

The practicalities

The essential practicalities in preparation are as follows.

Check the case details thoroughly and make sure you have all information and results to hand. Take the notes with you in case you need to refer to them for a detail. Remember that another member of staff present is helpful, not only for you but also to help and support relatives.

Your appearance is important. Is your white coat really necessary for this? If you must wear it, it should go without saying that you should make sure there are no blood stains, particularly if it is a case of major trauma.

Find a suitable private room, furniture arranged, tissues to hand, and make sure that you will be undisturbed. Make sure you allow yourself and the relatives time. Adopting an appropriate mood can be difficult if one is pressed for time, stressed or unprepared. Check identities and relationships, as it is not the time to get names and relationships wrong. Offer your own identity and status and that of anyone with you.

A brief, neutral conversation to establish rapport may be beneficial but should not delay getting on with the purpose of the meeting. You might explain why you have brought someone with you. The reason for the meeting should be explained. It is helpful to find out what they already know or have been told and it cannot be assumed they have previously been prepared for the possibility. Empathise, comfort where necessary, allow time for information to sink in, do not argue and allow relatives their expressions of anger without criticism. Check their understanding, invite questions and try to be practical.

Finally, offer to remain with them for a while in case they wish to ask questions, although they may wish to be alone. When finished, summarise and check what the relatives wish to do immediately. They may wish to see the body. Give them the opportunity to attend to their appearance if they have been crying. Ensure they are accompanied by a suitably trained member of staff.

Action

Ask if you can sit in with someone who is experienced and skilled at breaking bad news.

When you feel confident enough try doing it yourself, maybe with a more experienced person sitting in to help if things get difficult.

Afterwards reflect on what went well and what went less well, and ask for some feedback from the person who sat in to help.

Only when you feel confident, try doing these interviews on your own.

Children and bereavement

Children who are forewarned of the imminence and inevitability of death have lower anxiety levels as a result, compared with those who are not forewarned. Young children are often said to need the concrete experience of seeing the parent after death. The bereaved adult may find this difficult and the doctor may be able to offer to accompany the child. Further counselling is normally the responsibility of the primary care team, using appropriate counselling services as required. CRUSE – the national charity for bereavement care – publishes literature for bereaved children and their carers as well as providing training and counselling services.

For those requiring more on this subject please refer to the related reading at the end of this chapter.

Death and religion

Behaviour which is in ignorance of the religious beliefs and needs of a dying patient and their relatives may cause great distress and offence. These problems are most likely to occur when dealing with patients whose cultures and beliefs differ considerably from those of your own.

We will cover most of the main religions. It is also worth mentioning that there may be wide variations in Hinduism, Sikhism and Islam, depending on the country of origin or sect, particularly within the Indian subcontinent, and also differences between people from East Africa and those who have come from the Indian subcontinent. We have not tried to cover all aspects of these religions.

In many Eastern cultures, grief is often shown more openly than in the West, and wherever possible a side ward for the dying patient is helpful. Jewellery and insignia of possible religious significance should not be removed from the body without the permission of the relatives.

Buddhism

Buddhism was founded in the Indian subcontinent about 2500 years ago by an Indian prince, Siddartha Gautama. He tried to help his people find happiness and contentment by searching for truth. Sitting on a river bank under a sacred fig tree Gautama discovered four truths and from that point he was called Buddha. It is unique among the religions in acknowledging no single god as creator, but many gods, those lesser beings than Buddha himself. Some scholars argue that it is more a way of living than a true religion. There are two major schools of Buddhism and their attitudes differ in various ways. Although relief of pain and suffering are important, Buddhists often do not wish to have a clouded mind and may therefore be reluctant to take strong analgesics. They also tend to accept death relatively easily, looking forward to the next life with equanimity. After death the body must be wrapped in a sheet without emblems. There is usually a cremation conducted by a member of the family or a Buddhist bhikku or sister. There is a general calmness and acceptance of death by Buddhists.

Chinese religions

A popular Chinese saying states 'three religions – one religion' or 'three paths to the same goal'. Basically the Chinese religious experience finds philosophical expression in a fusion of Confucianism, Taoism and Buddhism. Even Chinese Christians practise some rituals that are Buddhist or Taoist.

Central to all Chinese religion is the family and belief in ancestors. An impending death is accepted as a natural event. Coffins are often purchased earlier in life. A dying person may even have their coffin in the room with them. Everything is done to convey to the dying person that they will be buried properly, with dignity and pomp. Concern for the propriety after death is universal.

After death the body is washed by the family an uneven number of times in special water thought to be protected by a guardian spirit. Before being dressed the body is covered in wadding, also to keep the evil spirits out. The garments have no buttons or zips but fabric ties. Burial is normal. Death and dying are the culmination of the religious life of Chinese people and a proper funeral is of great importance. The dying person will want to know (and may seek reassurance) that these things will be carried out correctly.

Christianity

Christians believe that Jesus was the son of God. There are many branches of Christianity with varying emphases. They all believe in an afterlife but concepts of this vary.

The three main divisions behave differently at the time of death. The orthodox Christian may request a bible, crucifix and a prayer book, and before death the priest may be asked to visit the patient. The priest may hear a last confession, anoint the patient with oil or give communion. Christians are usually buried and there are no restrictions about handling the body.

Roman Catholics believe the Pope is the spiritual successor to Saint Peter. Roman Catholics tend to be regular church-goers and so a bedside service by the parish priest or Roman Catholic hospital chaplain is important. When the patient is dying the priest will minister the 'sacrament of the sick', popularly known as 'the last rites'. The family may ask for the patient's hands to be placed in an attitude of prayer, holding a crucifix or rosary. There are no restrictions about handling the body.

Protestant Christianity developed during the sixteenth century. The Church of England maintains the traditional order of priests and bishops. The Free Church and the Church of Scotland have different practices. Generally Protestants have fewer last rites. Some patients may ask for a last communion.

Quakers (The Religious Society of Friends) have no clergy, but the presence of another Quaker or the hospital chaplain is usually acceptable. Burials in other groups, such as Plymouth Brethren, Jehovah's Witnesses and Mormons, normally follow customary Christian practice. With these it is sensible to ask a family member for advice.

Hinduism

Hindus believe in a supreme being residing in the individual, the ultimate goal being the release of the individual's soul from the cycle of birth, death and rebirth to join the supreme being. A person's deeds in their past lives determine status and good or ill fortune in the present life, whose quality, in turn, governs future lives.

There is no supreme church authority and no hierarchy. Numerous gods are worshipped, each being the personification of a particular aspect of the supreme being. Most families worship at a shrine in their home, attending the temple only for communal worship. The temple is in the care of a priest, who is generally a member of the highest caste, chosen and supported by the community. The priest has no parochial functions, but may come to the hospital to pray with the relatives of a dying person. When death is thought to be near, a family member or priest reads from one of the holy books of Hinduism. Many Hindu patients prefer to die at home and this should be respected whenever possible.

Normally the family wish is to wash and lay out the body. This may be done at home or at the undertakers. The body is generally covered with a plain white sheet, though married Hindu women are often shrouded in red. The priest may tie a thread round the neck or wrist and this should not be removed. After death, gloves should be worn by non-Hindus when touching or moving the body.

The eldest son is generally responsible for making the funeral arrangements. All Hindus, except stillborn babies and very young children, are usually cremated. Although in India this would be done on the day of death, in Britain this is impracticable. Post-mortems are not generally approved of, but if legally required by a coroner they are accepted, provided the situation is fully explained. There are no religious prohibitions against the giving or receiving of organs. The family is in mourning until the thirteenth day following cremation, when a special ceremony takes place.

Islam

'Islam' means submission (to the will of God). A Muslim is a follower of Islam. Muslims believe in one god (Allah), and that Mohammed, who was born in 570AD in Mecca, was his prophet or messenger. Mohammed is regarded as the last of a long line of prophets including Abraham, Moses, David, Job, John the Baptist and Jesus. The Koran consists of the word of God as told by Mohammed and this, together with his recorded sayings and acts, constitutes the Islamic legal system. Muslims believe in life after death and that a person will be judged by God according to his deeds and sent to heaven or to hell.

The mosque is the centre for worship and is in the charge of an imam who is elected and supported by the congregation. The imam is not required to attend the death of a Muslim or to officiate at a burial, but is usually invited to do so.

The family prays at the bedside of the dying person, whose head must be turned towards Mecca, which may entail altering the position of the bed. The call to prayer is whispered into his ear. Normally family members wash and lay out the body, either in the mortuary or at the undertakers. Non-Muslims touching the body must wear gloves.

Muslims are buried, never cremated. Women never go to the funeral. Burial should take place as soon after death as possible. It is not always possible in Britain to comply strictly with all the Islamic rules for burial, so some families take their dead back to their country of origin. This entails much bureaucratic delay which is very distressing to the relatives but it is also the Islamic ideal to be buried in one's 'homeland'. The bereaved family are in mourning for three days after the funeral and visit the grave every Friday during the following 40 days.

As the body must not be cut or defaced, routine post-mortems are never accepted. Coroner's cases are reluctantly accepted if the circumstances are explained to the relatives and safeguards are given that organs will not be removed. Organ donation and transplant requests are rarely allowed, but there is variation in practice. Refusal should not be assumed.

Judaism

Jews regard Abraham as the founder of Judaism. Even for the least religious Jew, there is a strong sense of the value of human life, derived from the idea of God creating man in his own image. But it also means that doctors and other healthcare professionals are often highly respected by Jews, so religious laws can be broken in order to save or preserve life. Indeed there are strict laws on preserving life. This attitude may make Jews less good at dealing with death and the dying, although they are very good at looking after the bereaved, giving them comfort and support. Although the dying patient may wish to see a Rabbi there are no last rites. Hospital staff who call a Rabbi will also need to know whether the patient is orthodox or reform (liberal).

Traditionally, the first acts after death, of shutting the eyes and laying the arms straight, are done by members of the family or other Jews, although in hospital this may not be possible. With this in mind, the Sexton's office of the United Synagogue Burial Society issued guidelines in 1960 for handling the bodies of Jews after death.

Orthodox and some non-orthodox Jews continue a custom of having watchers who stay with the body day and night, reciting Psalms, although this is not usually for long because Jews expect to bury their dead as quickly as possible.

Post-mortems, unless required by law, are forbidden by orthodox Jews and the donation of organs except corneas is frowned upon. Reform, liberal or non-observant Jews are more relaxed about this. For the orthodox, the body will be removed and all washing carried out as a ritual of purification. Burial in a Jewish cemetery is the only option for an orthodox Jew.

After the burial there is a formal period of mourning for seven days when the bereaved stay at home and receive friends, relatives and visitors who come to pay their respects and show sympathy and support – an example of the strong emphasis on supporting the living.

Sikhism

The word Sikh means disciple or follower. The Sikh religion was founded in the sixteenth century by a Hindu, Guru Nanak, who rebelled against various aspects of Hinduism. Sikhs believe in one god, and Guru Nanak is revered as a man chosen by God to reveal his message. In Sikhism men and women are equal. There are no ordained priests and the Sikh temple is in the care of a reader who is appointed and supported by the community.

When a person is close to death, the family, sometimes accompanied by the priest, pray at the bedside and read from the holy book. Sikhs have no objection to the body being touched by non-Sikhs, although family members usually lay out and wash the body themselves. The body is taken to the undertakers by way of the family home, where the coffin is opened so that the dead person may be seen for the last time. All Sikh men and women, in life and after death, must wear the five signs of Sikhism: uncut hair (and beard); a semicircular comb which fixes the uncut hair in a bun; a steel or occasionally gold bangle worn on the right wrist; a symbolic dagger worn under the clothes in a small cloth sheath or simply as a shaped brooch or pendant; and long undershorts reaching to the knees, now often replaced by ordinary underpants which have the same significance. Sikh men wear their turban after death. All Sikhs, apart from stillborn babies and infants dying within a few days of birth, are cremated.

There is no religious objection to post-mortem, but there may be some resistance to the idea from families originating in rural areas. Requests for organ transplantation are acceptable. The family is in mourning for about ten days, though this varies.

Helping or counselling

Nursing staff are helpful in advising bereaved relatives on the procedures for registration of death, cremation certificates and finding a suitable undertaker. The hospital chaplain may take on these duties and therefore be able to put relatives in touch with members of their own religion or community when no relatives are easily accessible.

Requesting a post-mortem

There are two possible reasons for requesting a post-mortem. The first arises as a statutory requirement if a coroner's inquest is to be held. The second occurs when it is felt significant benefit would be gained from further investigation into the cause of death.

Some communication skills (such as the breaking of bad news) are transferable between different areas of clinical practice. Autopsy requests represent a specific application for communication skills training that is probably not directly transferable and therefore requires specific attention.

Clinicians with little or no interest in autopsies may still have to inform relatives of the requirement for a medico-legal autopsy. All clinicians should therefore be capable of providing adequate reassurance to bereaved relatives regarding the autopsy. Clinicians who cannot provide adequate reassurance regarding the fears and reservations expressed by relatives are often reluctant to request autopsies because of the personal discomfort experienced when approaching bereaved relatives for consent.

The process of requesting an autopsy from recently bereaved relatives is stressful for doctors and any sense of personal discomfort will decrease the motivation of clinicians to request autopsies. This difficult request of relatives often falls to junior staff. A request for a post-mortem is of necessity made at a time of grief and distress for relatives, especially as they tend to be associated with a bereavement that was sudden, unexpected or traumatic. There is likely therefore to be denial and perhaps dissociation in addition to the grief. The relatives' mental state may thus understandably be difficult to deal with and you may encounter anger, resentment or rejection.

Many studies have highlighted the problems of obtaining permissions for autopsies and yet most clinicians have had no formal training in the matter. Studies have also shown how provision of training in requesting permission for autopsies has contributed to the improvement in autopsy rates. Those clinicians who have received appropriate training have more confidence and consequently may be more willing to take the time to educate relatives in the nature and importance of the autopsy. The manner in which permission for autopsy is sought is thus important and can in some cases influence the decision of the family.

Although formal training is thought to be appropriate between the beginning of the final undergraduate year and the end of the pre-registration house officer year, some further assistance is useful later on. Active methods, such as demonstration video sessions, video feedback sessions based on the performance of participants and role–play techniques, have all been found to be more desirable than the more passive training methods, such as written guidelines and lectures. Your local trust may well provide such opportunities.

It may be better to break the bad news separately from gaining permission for a post-mortem. You also need to agree on who is going to do it and who you will ask for permission.

Key people involved with agreeing post-mortems

The doctor

Breaking bad news is difficult enough for any doctor – having to deal with distressed relatives and give bad news is a significant stress for all doctors. Being less experienced and less senior adds to that stress and the difficulty of requesting a post-mortem adds even further to the stress.

It is easy to think that your main task is to get permission. But that takes account neither of your personal attitude to dying, death and post-mortem examinations, nor your feelings about what a post-mortem may say of the correct diagnosis, possibly revealing errors in earlier diagnosis and treatment.

Family members

In the emotionally charged atmosphere it is also easy to forget that the family are likely to want an answer too, not for any reason of possible litigation, but in the natural desire to know why, what happened and how.

Relatives will have personal, religious and cultural attitudes towards death and medical science. They may have a fear about the body being cut up or that their relative may not really be dead. A poorly handled request for a post-mortem can be a source of additional stress to relatives.

The pathologist

This is not a two-party process but a triangle, with the person carrying out the post-mortem involved. It is easy for them to forget about their colleagues who have to discuss issues face-to-face with relatives. Delays in getting results to medical staff can be frustrating, contribute to tensions and cause worry. For relatives, delays can be agonising.

The approach

Some individual doctors' approaches can be helpful and soften the blow, whereas others may exacerbate the emotional trauma for relatives. Relatives seem to gain support when they perceive that the informant is also distressed. A cold, impersonal, 'professional' approach might even cause offence. There are basically three ways of approaching the problem:

• blunt and insensitive, accepting that relatives will be upset whatever is said
• kind and sad but without any positive support, encouragement or optimism
• understanding and positive, with flexibility, reassurance and empathy.

The right approach is obvious, but you will be aware that there are many complicating factors, most of which we hope we have covered in the preceding sections.

Making the request for a post-mortem

In olden times, messengers bringing news of battles lost were often executed. There is still a tendency to blame a messenger for bad news and doctors are no exception. Patients, and doctors too, often harbour unrealistic expectations of modern medicine. The guidelines for breaking bad news are relevant here (*see* p. 101).

People respond according to their personality, which is often difficult to predict. Stunned silence, disbelief, guilt, anger and acute stress can all occur. Anger and acute stress are especially problematic, but stunned silence and disbelief are also difficult. Anger may be directed at the doctor, the medical profession, medical science, the hospital or at the NHS in general, but meeting this with anger, or defensively, only exacerbates the situation.

Allowing relatives to cry can be important for them. People value doctors who can cope with tears without getting embarrassed. The doctor's instinctive reaction is usually to treat tears like haemorrhage – stop them as quickly as possible. Doctors should be able to display emotion, particularly as professional detachment can so easily be interpreted as evasive and unsympathetic.

Remember that the most difficult aspects for the clinician are unlikely to be of any concern to the relative, so it is important to check continually on the responses and feelings of a relative, allowing the time and opportunity for things to sink in and to answer any questions.

Reporting cases to the coroner

The coroner's officers must be informed of all reportable deaths. These are categorised in instructions to Registrars of Deaths, but the cases you are likely to be involved with would include the following.

Deaths in hospital:

- within 24 hours of admission
- during an operation
- before recovery from anaesthetic
- within 24 hours of leaving theatre.

In addition there are cases which you might experience in A & E and which usually result in an inquest. They are generally non-natural causes of death and are as follows:

- cause unknown
- has occurred in suspicious circumstances
- due to violence or neglect
- due to an accident, whether at home, at work or any other situation
- has occurred in prison or police custody
- alcoholic poisoning
- drug poisoning
- abortion
- stillbirth if there is any reason to believe that the child was born alive
- industrial disease or poisoning
- septicaemia associated with an injury or industrial disease.

Cases relating to violence or injury are still reportable even later, when death occurs less than a year and a day after the event causing the injury. An injury includes burns, choking, fractures (pathological fractures are usually excluded), foreign bodies, concussion, cuts, drowning, hyperthermia and hypothermia, sunstroke, lightning, electric shock, etc.

Unless it is clear that death is due to a known natural cause it will normally be necessary for a post-mortem examination to be carried out. The permission of the relatives is not needed but they of course must be informed and notified of the time and place, unless this would unduly delay the examination. The relatives and other recognised persons are entitled to be represented at the post-mortem examination by a medical practitioner.

Action

Check out the written guidelines your hospital has for reporting cases to the coroner.

At an inquest

Appearances in court are rare and in spite of the increase in litigation, the number of negligence cases that reach court is still very small. A far more likely appearance is in the coroner's court at an inquest. This can still have implications for your reputation.

Definitions

A coroner is an independent judicial officer of the Crown whose duties are assigned under the *Statute of the Coroners' Act* 1988. The coroner investigates the circumstances of certain deaths and must be a registered medical practitioner, barrister or solicitor of a least five years' standing. Each year in the UK about 180 000 cases are reported to a coroner and over half of these are by doctors. An inquest is a fact-finding enquiry to establish who died where, when and how, and the cause of death.

There will normally be guidelines written for your trust, particularly for dealing with cases that may have implications for the reputation of the hospital or the staff, especially in cases in which there may be media interest. Trusts normally provide appropriate managerial, legal and personal support.

Giving evidence

Careful preparation and familiarity with the events of the case are important. Witnesses are generally put at ease and the procedure is more informal than in other courts. Witnesses still take an oath or affirm. Each witness is taken through their statement by the coroner and questions asked where necessary. Family or their representatives may then ask questions. When the family is unhappy or angry they may have legal representation.

The normal approach to dealing with legal decisions in English courts is by adversarial debate. Coroner's inquests are different. This is an inquiry, not adversarial, so coroners will not usually tolerate hostile questioning of witnesses. Where there is disagreement between witnesses the coroner will hear all evidence and the evidence thus presented enables the coroner to reach a verdict. Solicitors may view an inquest as a preliminary investigation to a claim, but it is not for the coroner to apportion blame or deal with matters of negligence or civil liability.

Solicitors often advise witnesses to follow three 'golden rules':

- dress up
- speak up
- shut up!

So it is sensible to dress for the occasion, to take notes with you to refer to, having rehearsed them so that you can deliver your message with confidence, and, when you have said what you planned to say, sit down as soon as you have given simple answers to any questions. Do not dig a hole for yourself. If you do not know the answer, say so. Speculation or trying to be helpful is a pitfall to avoid.

Summing up and conclusions

The coroner will sum up the findings and conclusions and the verdict will comprise:

- name of the deceased
- illness or injury that caused death
- the time, place and circumstances in which the injury or illness was sustained
- coroner's conclusion as to cause of death
- registration particulars.

The coroner's rules allow no verdict to be framed in a way that appears to determine criminal or civil liability. Inevitably, the verdict that gives rise to most concern is 'lack of care'. The court of appeal has recommended that this is replaced by 'to which neglect contributed'.

The duty of confidentiality does not end with the patient's death. After the inquest there may be questions from the press. It is acceptable and courteous to convey, publicly to the family, sympathy at the death and distress. It is not appropriate without the consent of family to volunteer further information. Never talk to the press without professional guidance.

In a trust it is usual for an individual to be designated the task of co-ordinating the gathering of information and providing this for the coroner. The report should be factual and accurate. You should refresh your memory as to the sequence of events using medical records, which are an essential part of the investigation. Avoid technical language and detailed explanation of complex procedures. Times of events should be given as precisely as possible. An account of the practitioner's personal involvement should be in sequence. Other staff should be identified so that their comments can be sought where necessary.

Action

If you have time, why not go and see an inquest. A call to the coroner's office will tell you when the next ones are booked.

Complaints

Complaints fall into three main areas.

- Complaints, whether clinical or non-clinical, made against you or the hospital by dissatisfied patients and relatives with whom you have direct contact.
- Complaints about the whole team, medical outcomes, administrative and support service, and the hospital generally. These can be made by patients and relatives or organisations representing patients' interests.
- Internal employee complaints made against the hospital.

Employment complaints are normally the subject of internal trust procedures and are monitored by the personnel department. If you do become involved in a complaint related to employment we suggest you contact the local BMA office and seek the advice of the industrial relations officer.

Dealing with an informal patient complaint

Complaints are usually due to one or more of the following:

- perceived failure of the doctor to deliver an expected standard of care
- unrealistic expectation of the patient or relatives
- failure of communication.

A complaint is not a claim, but it could become one. It is important that it should be handled well. Usually this means a prompt explanation to any patient or their relative involved in any event that has given rise to the complaint. Minor criticism should be dealt with by conciliation not confrontation. Deal with the situation sympathetically. An apology can be given, as an apology is not an admission of legal liability.

When you find yourself first in line when a patient or relative complains, it is helpful to remember that the complainant is usually angry so:

- try to be on a level with the other person – if you are looking down on them they may feel more threatened
- allow them plenty of personal space and do not get too close as this could also make them feel threatened
- acknowledge the other's feelings by an empathic statement – the other person now understanding that you understand means they no longer have to prove their anger
- indicate that you are listening by reflective listening, repeating back a summary of what is being said
- avoid questioning an angry person
- if you are in a closed space or room check that you are well positioned for leaving quickly, or at least ensure that a large piece of furniture separates you from the complainant!

Use simple assertiveness techniques (*see* p. 36 on assertiveness) such as the 'broken record' to express yourself calmly and persistently as the angry person often leaps from topic to topic.

They may use criticism as a weapon, so again use the 'broken record'. It can be helpful to use another assertiveness technique called 'fogging'. This is simply a method of taking the wind out of your critic's sails by saying that there may be some truth in what they are saying or agreeing in principle with them.

Formal complaints procedures

More serious complaints should be reported and handled by formal procedures as they may lead to a claim for compensation. These should be referred to a person of sufficient seniority for advice and for them to deal with the situation as required. Most trusts have well-documented procedures for handling complaints and these should always be followed.

NHS complaints procedure

From 1 April 1996, a new procedure for dealing with complaints about NHS services was introduced. This followed a review by an independent committee chaired by Professor Alan Wilson, Vice-Chancellor of Leeds University. There are two elements to the new system (local resolution and independent review), both of which should be managed by an appropriate person.

Local resolution

This involves the provider of the service trying to resolve the complaint to the patient's satisfaction – in the majority of cases on an informal basis – as quickly as possible. Your trust is certain to have written guidelines on its complaints procedure. As a first step, complaints should receive a response immediately or within a specified timescale. Oral responses initally, supported by a written response. This may include the offer of investigation or conciliation if appropriate.

The clinical director, department head or complaints officer then follows this up, either orally or in writing, within a period of 21 to 28 days. *The Patient's Charter* gives the complainant the right to receive a full and prompt written reply to a formal complaint from the chief executive. In particularly serious cases or where the complainant remains dissatisfied, the investigation may well need to be detailed and may include obtaining independent advice. Complainants also have to be made aware of both the role of the Community Health Council (CHC) and any patient's advocate available (and how they may be contacted) to assist them in pursuing their complaints.

Most dissatisfied patients require explanations or apologies for poor service and assurances that defects will be remedied, rather than financial compensation. Only a relatively small number of complaints proceed to litigation in the end.

Independent review

If local resolution fails, the complainant can seek a further review of the complaint by a convenor (normally a non-executive director of the trust or health authority concerned) who will be advised by an independent lay person. If the convenor decides that more could be done to satisfy the complainant, they may either establish an independent panel to consider the complaint or ask the service provider to take further local resolution action. The complaint will be referred on to the health service commissioner (ombudsman) if the complainant is dissatisfied with the response from the NHS.

Health service commissioner (ombudsman)

The ombudsman has the power to investigate written complaints from the public about the provision of services or maladministration. The commission has the power to examine internal papers and clinical records. Any doctor faced with a request to give a report should take advice.

Complainants who remain dissatisfied after the NHS complaints procedure has been completed, may ask the ombudsman to investigate their case. The ombudsman is completely independent of the NHS and of government, and can consider complaints about most aspects of NHS services and treatment. However, he is not obliged to investigate every complaint put to him.

Roles of parties to a complaint

There may be any number of parties involved in a complaint. The following is a summary of those who might be involved, and some aspects of their roles.

Patient's advocate

If the complainant is not the patient, it is important to be clear just what the nature of the complaint is and the complainant's perspective: is the complainant acting on behalf of the patient? If so, do they have the authority of the patient to do so.

Patient's family or carers

It should be established whether the complainant is acting on behalf of a wider group or drawing upon a wider knowledge base than is immediately obvious.

Complaints manager

Trusts and health authorities must have a designated complaints manager who is readily accessible to the public and is directly accountable to the chief executive. In general practice this might be a senior partner or practice manager

Convenor

The convenor is a non-executive director appointed by the board to manage the independent review panel process. Where a complaint relates in whole, or in part, to action taken in exercising clinical judgement, the convenor must take appropriate clinical advice.

Community Health Council (CHC)

The CHC may be involved at an early stage or brought in when the complainant is not happy with the initial response. The CHC may act as advocate for the complainant. (*See* p. 178 for changes to CHCs.)

Healthcare professionals

A complaint can harm a professional's career, especially if poorly handled. To ensure they do not feel excluded from the process, they normally draft the response that will go to the complainant. If an apology is required, this can be the clinician's own letter with a follow-up by the chief executive, thus ensuring compliance with the regulations.

Professional bodies

Allowances are made in the planning for the involvement of a professional's representative body. The representative body can also provide independent support to a professional.

Health authority or other purchasers

Contractual requirements with health authorities or GP fundholders may place different and possibly conflicting obligations concerning complaints recording and reporting. The organisation's complaints procedure should meet all these requirements.

Trade unions

Trade unions or other staff bodies will be interested in the complaints procedure and likely to play an active part in supporting its members.

The media

The NHS is a popular topic for both local and national media. The episode may come under media scrutiny. Some letters may appear in the press if the complainant is unhappy.

The board

Complaints have to be reported to the board quarterly. The board has to produce an annual report on complaints handling, and circulate it widely.

Health service commissioner (ombudsman)

If a complainant is not successful in getting an independent review panel established, or is unhappy with the outcome of the panel, then he or she can approach the ombudsman.

Action

Look at the summary document of your trust's complaints procedure.

Related reading

Buckman R (1992) *How to Break Bad News: a guide of health care professionals*. Johns Hopkins University Press, Baltimore.

DHSS (1990) *Informed Consent*, HC(90)22. HMSO, London.

DoH (1992) *NHS Guidelines – patients who die in hospital* HSG(92). DoH, London.

Dyregrow A (1991) *Grief in Childhood: a handbook for adults*. Jessica Kingsley, London.

Evans J (1999) *Clinical Negligence in NHS and the Law*. Wellard's NHS Handbook 1999/2000.

Faulkner A (1998) *When the News is Bad: a guide for health professionals*. Stanley Thornes, Cheltenham.

Gillon R (1985) Telling the truth and medical ethics. *BMJ*. **291**: 1556–7.

Heegaard M (1991) *When Someone Very Special Dies: children can learn to cope with grief*. Woodland, Minneapolis.

Heegaard M (1991) *When Something Terrible Happens: children can learn to cope with grief*. Woodland, Minneapolis.

Neuberger J (1991) *Caring for Dying People of Different Faiths* (2e). Mosby, London.

NHSE (1990) *A Guide to Consent for Examination*. NHSE, London.

Vincent C (ed) (1995) *Clinical Risk Management*. BMJ Publishing Group, London.

5

Teaching, training, appraisal and assessment

This chapter aims to help you make the most of your structured learning opportunities as an SpR, to provide you with the 'tools' to support others, and to help them learn from you. It also addresses the important areas of revalidation, appraisal and assessment.

Teaching and training

SpRs are both undergoing training and providing it for the benefit of others. Their continuing medical and professional development is critical to career success and to safe and effective delivery of service to patients. The training of SpRs is laid down by the Calman Implementation Steering Group and is the subject of a training agreement. The following chapter provides an insight into all aspects of your training responsibilities as an SpR.

Differences between competence and confidence, and between teaching and training

Experience by itself is insufficient to develop competence. There is evidence to suggest that confidence levels (but not skill levels) grow with experience alone (Marteau *et al.* 1990). Feedback on performance, combined with an unflagging commitment to learning, are prerequisites for continuing professional development. This feedback comes from other, usually more senior, colleagues. This is often referred to as teaching or training. There is some confusion about the meaning of the terms 'teaching' and 'training'. We will employ definitions for the purposes of this handbook which are outlined below (*see* pp. 123–4), although you will hear them used in many differing contexts in everyday language.

We tend to think of learning as a formal process, although much real learning is informal. It occurs on a day-to-day basis without our being particularly aware of it. We discussed this process in Chapter 1. The choice of method of delivery is often made according to the needs and preferences of the teacher rather than the needs of learners. This is a pity, because it can lead to much time wasting for those involved. A better basis would be the choice of opportunities available and the nature, or learning domains, of the material to be learnt.

Learning domains

The nature of the task to be learnt can vary in content and complexity which can influence the approach to teaching. The following categorisation of learning situations represents a simple way of helping to decide which approach to teaching is likely to be most helpful to the learner.

Understanding

This is usually acquired as knowledge grows, concepts are grasped and, eventually, learners are able to put together the whole picture for themselves. Often described as the 'cognitive domain', understanding may be developed through reading, studying, question and answer and discussion sessions. Highly developed understanding enables the learner to apply the learning by undertaking an analysis of complex cases, deriving solutions and evaluating outcomes.

Skills

Practical skills, sometimes referred to as being in the 'psychomotor domain', are those that usually involve practice in order to acquire full competence. Learning is achieved through instruction and guided practice. This is what we have referred to as training. Instruction may be as short as three or four minutes and usually takes place during normal working. Adult learners usually find periods of skills training of more than about 15 minutes to be difficult. They generally want to be involved and begin to practise newly learned skills.

Other, more complex, skills are employed when dealing with people. These might be colleagues or patients, individuals or groups. Interpersonal skills are of considerable importance in teamwork, including handling conflict, influencing, counselling and information gathering. They can also enable you to get important information from patients to aid diagnosis. Such skills are more difficult to impart. Demonstration, role-playing and feedback using video can be helpful. Again, guided practice is an effective way of following up initial training. Professionals frequently find it difficult to admit, even to themselves, that they need help in dealing with others. Most of us believe we are good at communicating. Recognising your need is the first stage in learning.

Attitudes

Attitudes are usually described as being in the 'affective domain' and are based on complex sets of values and beliefs. These are acquired throughout life and are dependent on a wide range of influences. The most important influences are usually close contacts such as family, friends and significant work colleagues. 'Role models' are often referred to in the training of professionals. Affective development is partly dependent on the influence of those who impress us during our formative learning stages. Senior colleagues have almost certainly influenced your attitudes to many aspects of your work, perhaps even your choice of career. You, in turn, will help to shape the attitudes of more junior colleagues. Indeed, you may also help shape the attitudes of some of your senior colleagues.

Teaching and training require developed skills. The following text will help you to understand how to do it, but there is no substitute for guided practice. Every time you help others to learn, try to get feedback on your own performance.

Teaching

Teaching is taken to describe pre-arranged situations in which one person delivers learning material to a group, normally as a formal presentation. Such sessions can take place within the hospital or off-site, according to the demands of the learning. They usually concentrate on one-way transfer of information, rather then the passing on of skills. The presentation may be in the form of a tutor-led discussion or a lecture – the latter has been described as an activity during which the notes of the lecturer are transferred to the notebooks of the students without passing through the minds of either! Good teachers can generally make their presentations interesting and sufficiently relevant to avoid this description.

Teaching is a didactic process which focuses on formal presentations such as lectures, where the communication is mainly one way. Please refer to Chapter 3 of this handbook for a detailed guide to presentation techniques.

The defining characteristic of a teaching session is the expectation (or hope, at least) that the audience will leave with an improved level of understanding of the topic, and perhaps be able to develop their own capability as a result. Your first responsibility, then, is to select, arrange and deliver your material to meet their expectations. It is helpful to start by attempting to define the needs of the audience – rather than first deciding what you want to tell them.

The next responsibility is to find and use ways of making your delivery interesting as well as relevant. Personal skills in delivery can be developed, either through attending a training course or by practising and getting feedback from reliable members of your audiences. Sensible use of audio-visual aids, careful planning and, when possible, audience participation will help to create effective teaching sessions.

Training

Training or instruction is a two-way process in which the learner is helped to develop their understanding and to practise a skill or set of skills. It is usually only through continuing practice that a satisfactory level of competence is achieved.

The focus here is on the development of skills in others. Practical skills are best trained on a one-to-one basis, where the learner can be involved in as much of the procedure as possible.

Each training event should be planned, and the following should be taken into account.

- *Current level of capability of the trainee.* This means checking that they are ready for the learning and that it fits with their current needs. By discussing their needs with them it is probable that their motivation to learn will also be increased.
- *Resources should be available to complete the whole training session.* These include your time, equipment, a room, other participants in the process – e.g. patients and any paperwork that is associated with the activity.
- *Learning goals or objectives for the session.* These should be agreed with the trainee and stated in measurable terms.
- *Method of instruction.* This is dealt with in more detail below.
- *Evaluation.* The criteria for success should have been determined, preferably by agreement with the trainee, before the instruction starts.
- *Record of completion.* It helps to record their achievement of the learning goals for their logbook.
- *Support and follow-up.* It is very important that learners are given time to master their new-found skills. They should not be left on their own without support and guidance being available during the early practice stages.

Method of instruction

The most common approach to skills training, and one which has stood the test of time, is the 'four-step' procedure. Most other methods of instruction are a variation on this theme. It helps to break down larger, more complex, tasks into smaller elements. The learner can be shown and can practise each separately before attempting the whole task as one.

- The trainer performs the task in the normal way with the learner observing. Questions should be saved until after the run-through.
- The trainer performs the task again while talking through each stage. There are three steps within this one – tell them what you are going to do – tell them while you are doing it – take time to deal with further questions after you have done it.
- The learner talks through the task while the trainer performs it. This gives the trainer an opportunity to check understanding.
- The learner performs the task and talks it through at the same time. Consolidation of learning begins at this stage. There is also the opportunity to stop the learner from making a mistake before it occurs. This is obviously critically important in some situations, e.g. in an operating theatre, where the learner would explain each step and get clearance from the trainer before proceeding.

Giving effective feedback is a key part of the training process. This is not always done as well as it should be. The following guidelines for giving feedback will help and they apply to most situations.

- *Maintain a positive approach.* Be encouraging and supportive.
- *Be direct.* Be specific and deal clearly with particular incidents and examples of behaviour. Avoid being woolly or vague.
- *Suspend judgement.* It is unhelpful to pronounce judgement but better to say how you see the situation and let the learner make their own evaluation.
- *Make it actionable.* It is not helpful to give someone feedback about something they cannot change. Useful feedback is that which can lead to a change in behaviour.
- *Time it well.* To be most effective it needs to be given as soon after the event as practical so it is fresh in the receiver's mind.

It would be an unusual learner who got everything right first time. You should always assume that learners will continue to need your support for some time after the training session is finished. At first this may involve direct supervision. Later they can be left alone to perform the task. Explain how you or some other suitable person can be contacted until the learner feels entirely sure of themselves.

Appraisal

Most doctors think firstly of appraisal as being focused on learners and related to the training process. In this case, it has been seen as developmental rather than judgemental. A well-conducted trainee appraisal meeting can provide an opportunity for the trainee to gain important new concrete experience through interaction with a senior colleague whose opinion is important to the trainee. The appraiser helps the trainee to reflect on experience and also assists in the acquisition and development of understanding of new concepts. It remains for the trainee to go out and test out their learning in their own way, taking action (under the supervision of a senior colleague) and acquiring new experience to reflect on later.

Appraisal has now been introduced for all doctors as part of the revalidation process. It thus contributes to a judgemental decision-making process. This type of appraisal, while still focusing on development, is also, in part at least, judgemental, in that the performance of the doctor will be assessed as part of the revalidation process. Evidence from appraisal forms part of the judgement.

Managers in the NHS are also appraised, usually on an annual basis. Managerial appraisal is used as a means of assessing performance, determining development needs and career advancement and, in some cases, pay awards. Figure 5.1 shows the relationships between the organisation's goals, the outside world, and the individual appraisal performance review process which is usually employed to monitor the performance of managers.

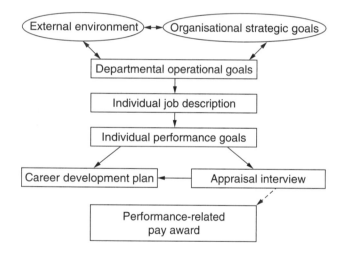

Figure 5.1 A typical managerial appraisal process.

Assessment

There are two types of assessment which overlap in definition with appraisal. The whole area is confused and we have tried here to make some sense of the language in use and the aims of the different approaches.

Formative assessment

Feedback on appraisal of performance which is primarily aimed at helping the appraisee to learn and develop is sometimes referred to as formative assessment. The Royal College of Obstetricians and Gynaecologists avoids using the word 'appraisal' – it instead uses the term 'formative assessment' to describe its equivalent to appraisal. This may be contrasted with summative assessment, which seeks to measure ability in order to make an award, or to permit progress over a performance hurdle such as in the annual assessment of SpRs. Similar terminology is used by the Royal College of General Practitioners, and elsewhere in healthcare education

Formative assessment is focused on the learner and educational needs. It attempts to measure skills, behaviours, attitudes or knowledge and may contain elements of self-assessment. Being assessed should encourage you to seek gaps and inform your educational plans. Finding weakness is positively encouraged as this offers learning opportunities.

The records of formative assessment are confidential to the parties involved and are usually held by the learner. The teacher's attitude should be non-judgemental and encourage the learners to explore themes that are unanticipated. Respect should be shown for the trainee by the contents of their learning plan being agreed through negotiation and openness, not coercion or manipulation.

Summative assessment

'Summative assessment' is the final, or end-of-year, criteria-based assessment introduced by Calman for the SpR grade. In addition to regular appraisal, SpRs are assessed each year in accordance with their Record of Individual (In-training) Training Assessment (RITA). The regulatory framework is set out in *A Guide to Specialist Registrar Training* (NHSE 1998). Difficulty sometimes arises for educational supervisors when deciding the extent to which they should regard the appraisal as confidential, particularly when the final RITA assessment report is to be prepared.

Summative assessment also tests for skills, behaviours, attitudes and knowledge, but is regulatory. The methods and criteria are set by examiners on behalf of an assessing body. Examiners themselves will have been trained in summative assessment methods. These need to be valid, reliable, feasible and fair. They can be either peer- or norm/criteria-referenced. For fairness, examinees should have access before the examination to the criteria by which they are being judged.

The aim of summative assessment is to identify those trainees who are not ready for independent practice. The results of summative assessment are not confidential. Outcomes will enhance or impede career progression.

Thus, there are four major types of appraisal or assessment. These, and their relationship with one another, are shown in Figure 5.2.

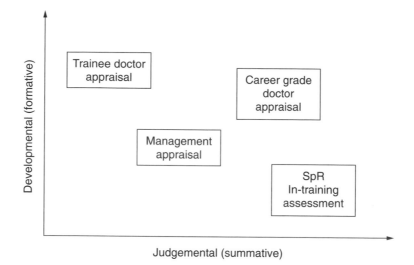

Figure 5.2 The relationship between appraisal and assessment systems used in the NHS.

The basic principles of assessment

- All require trust based on fairness and objectivity.
- Each type of assessment requires a different mixture of skills, knowledge and attitudes. Not all doctors will have the necessary skills and training to assess (or appraise) others.
- Doctors at the receiving end may also require training in how to prepare themselves and make the most of the experience.
- Those involved must know what type of process is being carried out.
- If a change from one type to another is required (e.g. when assessment moves into personal counselling), then permission must be sought.
- It should be clear to all parties whether an encounter is confidential or not.
- Some types of interaction do not sit well together, i.e. summative and formative assessment.

Although assessment is also part of the educational process it has an element of performance review. It is a process that is open and objective, subject to appeal and designed to inform decisions about career progress.

Managing the appraisal process

The main aim of this section is to provide a basis for successful medical appraisal interviews. Appraisal is an integral part of SpR training and has become a mandatory element in the revalidation process. Although the purpose of this book does not specifically require us to cover consultant appraisal for revalidation, the principles and suggested practice outlined below apply equally to most appraisal situations.

Trainee appraisal is a formative process. Although some judgement is involved, it is normally intended that the trainee should be developed, rather than assessed. Appraisal is intended to be part of the educational process. Kolb *et al.* (1984) proposed a model of learning which we explored in Chapter 1 (*see* Figure 1.2).

To repeat what was said on p. 125, a well-conducted appraisal meeting provides an opportunity for the trainee to gain important new concrete experience through interaction with a senior colleague whose opinion is important to the trainee. The appraiser helps the trainee to reflect on experience, and also assists in the acquisition and development of understanding of new concepts. It remains for the trainee to go out and test out the learning in their own way, taking risks (under the supervision of a senior colleague) and acquiring new experience to reflect on later.

Appraisal can:

- help identify educational needs at an early stage
- assist in the skills of self-reflection and self-appraisal that will be needed throughout a trainee's career
- enable learning opportunities that will be helpful to the trainee to be provided quickly
- provide a mechanism for reviewing progress and identifying problems in time for remedial action to be taken
- provide a mechanism for giving feedback on the quality of training provided
- make training more efficient and effective.

Appraisal meetings should take place at the beginning, halfway through and at the end of the post. The first meeting sets up the training agreement, which describes the learning objectives and confirms the support needed by the trainee during their time in the post. It is important that the trainee comes properly prepared for this meeting, and guidelines for this are given below. The second meeting is primarily concerned with reviewing progress, designing new learning opportunities if they are required and revising learning goals. The final meeting again reviews the trainee's experience, assists the trainee to reflect on experience gained, and helps to make sense of the complexities of the learning process. It will also, if required, address career-related issues. Appraisers should seek feedback from their trainees on the training and appraisal process at the end of every appraisal meeting.

Preparation for the appraisal meeting

As we indicated earlier, in your current role you may, at different times, be both appraiser and appraisee. First, we address the process for the appraisee.

Preparation: the trainee

You should be aware that the success of the appraisal meeting depends on adequate preparation by both parties. The list under *Preparing the agenda* (*see* p. 131) should help you to determine your most important topics. You should ask yourself the following questions, and take notes to the meeting:

Work performance
- Which areas of the work do you enjoy most?
- Which tasks do you feel you perform the best?
- Which areas do you find most challenging and why?
- How might you have improved your performance?

Skills/abilities
- Reflect on your strengths and weaknesses.
- Which skills do you have which you believe are well-developed?
- Identify those skills which need more development.

Learning objectives
- What learning objectives would you like to agree for the coming period of training?

Training
- Are there any specific training courses, or areas of need, which you would like to have addressed in the coming period?

Career
- What are the main career-related issues facing you at present? Are there still key decisions to be made? What help do you need with them?

Preparation: the appraiser

In your work as an SpR and, more significantly, as a consultant you are likely to be called upon to appraise colleagues. We concentrate here on the appraisal of trainees rather than colleagues. The aims of a trainee appraisal meeting are to identify relevant learning goals, to agree and commit to them, to reflect on and make sense of the trainee's past experience, and to agree and record actions based on the discussion. These might be for either the appraiser or trainee to implement.

The following guidelines are intended to enhance the quality of the appraisal for both parties.

- *Plan the meeting.* Dates and times for all meetings to be held during the post should be determined well in advance.
- *The trainee should be helped to prepare for the meeting.* After you have prepared an agenda you should show it to the trainee. The trainee preparation guidelines could be given to the trainee and discussed a few days before the meeting.
- *Relevant materials.* The curriculum, timetable, job description, rotas, previous appraisal records and notes of feedback from third parties should be collected together and considered before the meeting.
- *Suitable venue.* A quiet room, guaranteed free from interruptions, should be used. Bleeps and mobile phones must always be switched off or passed to a colleague.
- *Sufficient time.* There is no 'correct' amount of time to set aside for an appraisal meeting, but it is unlikely that much will be achieved in under half-an-hour. Note that the appraisal must take place in protected time.
- *Third parties.* Discuss the trainee with other consultants, trainees, nurses, midwives, technicians, physiotherapists or others as necessary to gain a rounded picture of the trainee.

Preparing the agenda

It helps if the pattern of the meeting is clear from the beginning for both parties. An agenda should be prepared and shared before the meeting. The following checklist should help you to prepare and conduct the appraisal. Choose from it the items you consider should make up the agenda for the meeting.

- *Education.* What, if any, examinations should be in preparation? What courses should be undertaken?
- *Academic/research.* Is advice necessary on research projects, or decisions to be made regarding suitable research designs?
- *Clinical experience and skills.* What specified procedures does the curriculum indicate? What levels of understanding and competence are indicated? Is good manual dexterity and hand/eye coordination necessary? Is experience of clinical risk management a requirement?
- *Knowledge.* What is an appropriate level of clinical knowledge? Is knowledge or use of evidence-based practice a requirement?
- *Organisation and planning.* What level of ability to organise their own work and

self-organisation are demanded of the trainee? Is active participation in audit an element of the training at this stage?

- *Teaching skills:*. Should the trainee be gaining experience of teaching others and, if so, at what level?
- *Career.* Should the trainee be helped to make career decisions at this stage? What help may be necessary? Would sharing your own experience be helpful to the trainee?
- *Personal skills and attributes.* The wide range of personal skills demanded in the work of a doctor is indicated below. Select those you feel should be discussed with the trainee:
  - *interpersonal communication*: rapport-building, listening, empathising, persuading and negotiating skills
  - *decisiveness*: taking responsibility, exerting appropriate authority
  - *teamworking*: cooperating with others, leading as required, seeking guidance
  - *flexibility and resilience*: able to adapt to rapidly changing circumstances and cope with setbacks
  - *thoroughness*: well-prepared, self-disciplined, punctual and committed to carry tasks through to completion
  - *drive and enthusiasm*: committed to patients and colleagues, motivated to achieve, curious, displaying initiative
  - *self-managed learning*: takes learning opportunities, reflects on experience, seeks guidance and advice
  - *probity*: honest, showing integrity and awareness of ethical dilemmas.
- *Feedback* from the trainee is usually helpful in enabling you to improve your approach.

Finally, the outcomes of the meeting should be recorded. It helps to remind you to include this stage by noting it in the agenda.

Conducting an appraisal meeting

The pattern of the meeting, partly determined by the level and experience of the trainee, should be dictated by the trainee's needs. Effective appraisal means getting the trainee to identify strengths and areas of need, and to propose ways of meeting the latter. Although guided by the appraiser, a successful meeting will feel as if it has been led by the trainee's priorities.

Confirm the agenda

The agenda should have been determined in advance with the trainee's help, but it is worthwhile briefly re-establishing the aims and key items for discussion. If a record of the previous appraisal is available, this should be used to inform the discussion at this stage.

Review past performance

Get the trainee talking as soon as possible. Use questions to open up issues and probe to help the trainee to explore their own strengths and weaknesses in the light of their performance. Try to avoid being directive. Allow the trainee to describe their perspective on issues and help them to reflect by using open and probing questions. Focus on specific aspects of the work. Give positive feedback where possible, particularly as a balance to any comments on less successful aspects of the trainee's work. Giving feedback requires a high level of skill and sensitivity. It demands a careful blend of drawing out the trainee to describe their own strengths and, particularly, weaknesses, and being direct in explaining concerns that you have, and that the trainee does not appear to recognise.

Explore and agree current learning needs

The trainee should have identified key learning needs in advance, but these may need to be modified in the light of the previous discussion. It may also be affected by information you have obtained from third parties in preparation for the meeting. You should remember that the responsibility for the trainee's learning is a joint one. Avoid taking on a list of jobs which could be more suitably undertaken by the trainee. Make brief notes to ensure you can recall critical issues. Reflect on learning objectives agreed for the post.

Agree learning objectives for the next period

These should be 'SMART'. This means they should be:

- **S**pecific – relate to specific tasks and activities, not general statements about improvement
- **M**easurable – it should be possible to assess whether or not it has been achieved
- **A**ttainable – given the time available, it should be possible for the trainee to achieve the desired outcome
- **R**ealistic – set within the trainee's capability
- **T**imed – the next appraisal date, or earlier, should be agreed as the time for reviewing the achievement of the objective.

Review and record decisions

You may wish to make brief notes throughout the meeting, in order to ensure that all the key points are reviewed at the end. It is vital that a record is kept of the outcome of the meeting. This should be agreed at the end of the meeting, and a copy kept by both parties. It will prove useful at the next meeting and may also form a useful document for the trainee to use as a record of progress in a logbook or portfolio. Doctors should retain records of appraisal meetings for their revalidation folders.

Get feedback on your performance

It is not common for appraisers to welcome informal feedback from the trainee at the end of an appraisal meeting. Indeed, it could prove to be an uncomfortable experience. Nevertheless, if the relationship between the two has developed positively, it can be very helpful for the appraiser to get an immediate indication of the benefits gained by the trainee. Bolder trainees may even give constructive criticism of the training received and any weaknesses perceived by them in the scheme. While this may be difficult, it will help future trainees and give the appraiser greater satisfaction in the long term. Alternatives include written feedback forms, which College tutors often use to route feedback to the Royal College.

Dealing with difficult issues

Confidentiality

There are mixed messages from some sources regarding the confidential nature of the appraisal meeting. Typically, it is suggested that if trainees are to feel free to express concerns about their capability or commitment to a specialty, then the appraiser must indicate that he or she will maintain confidentiality. On the other hand, in some cases the appraiser is also the assessor who is required to complete an assessment, in the case of SpRs, for the Record of Individual (In-training) Training Assessment (RITA). The final appraisal of pre-registration house officers is intended as the indicator of suitability for registration. In these and other cases, the appraiser/assessor is in a difficult situation if confidentiality is an issue. There may also be circumstances when the appraiser feels, in the interests of patient safety, that information about the trainee should be passed on to others.

Appraisers should help trainees to recognise that confidentiality is limited by the above conditions and that they will do all they can to support the trainee, while ensuring that the normal procedures are followed.

Conflict

The management of conflict has been addressed in Chapter 2. Disagreements are bound to arise from time to time and these should be resolved quickly to avoid escalation. Should serious conflict arise between an appraiser and trainee, it serves little purpose to attempt to resolve it since the trainee will always be concerned that fair assessment is compromised. A new appraiser should be found as quickly as possible.

Serious personal problems

Difficulties in appraisal may arise due to the serious nature of personal problems that afflict some trainees from time to time. It is important that the appraiser takes responsibility for ensuring the trainee receives suitable support in these circumstances. They should not, however, assume responsibility for taking on a counselling role or becoming personally burdened with the trainee's situation. Further advice on counselling is given below. Occupational health officers or personnel departments can usually assist in such circumstances.

Lack of personal insight

Occasionally, trainees seem to lack the ability to see their own weaknesses as others see them. This can be particularly true where there is a lack of interpersonal skill. It may also be that trainees are not able to see their lack of progress in developing clinical competence and judgement. It is important to distinguish between those who really are unaware of the negative impact they create or the concerns of other staff at the inadequacy of their clinical practice, and those who refuse to admit to weakness in order to protect themselves from negative consequences. In the latter case, it is important to help the trainee to recognise the value of talking about their problems, since it may lead to better career decisions if they are struggling with the demands of the specialty in which they are working. Once again, the most helpful way to do this is to use open and probing questions focused on specific examples of their performance to get them to confront the problem. Those trainees who truly are unable to see their weakness, even after supportive questioning and gentle challenge, will only perhaps come to terms with their situation when they fail an assessment. It is crucial that the clinical tutor, and perhaps the postgraduate dean, is made aware of such problems at as early a stage in training as possible.

Revalidation

It is relevant to touch briefly on revalidation here. Appraisal provides a basis for determining education and development plans. It also contributes to the revalidation process. The revalidation folder contains information on how well the doctor is practising and evidence of continuing professional development. Professional development portfolios are designed by the medical Royal Colleges and maintained by all doctors. These provide the evidence on which appraisal is based. Any concerns regarding a doctor's fitness to practise should be raised at the time of the appraisal. There should be no surprises at the revalidation stage. Thus, appraisal for revalidation is essentially similar to trainee appraisal. The major part addresses all aspects of performance and should relate to:

- good clinical care
- maintaining good practice
- relationship with patients
- working with colleagues
- teaching and training
- probity
- health.
  (*Source*: GMC 1997)

Preparation for appraisal relies heavily on the appraisee, who should have collected information about performance from a range of sources, including:

- patients – e.g. through a patient survey
- immediate colleagues such as partners or other professionals – e.g. through a peer-associate questionnaire
- managers, where appropriate
- colleagues who refer to, or accept referrals from, the doctor
- the doctor, e.g. through a self-assessment questionnaire.

Conducting a revalidation appraisal meeting

Peer appraisal can be a difficult and sensitive process. It is vital that discussion focuses on specific aspects of the appraisee's work, and avoids generalities that fail to address critical issues.

It is not normally the function of appraisal to deal directly with major problems, but merely to identify them and, ideally, to engage the appraisee in planning ways of addressing them. Revalidation guidelines emphasise the importance of dealing with problems locally as they arise (Gatrell and White 2000).

Supporting and advising others

Mentoring

In Greek mythology in *Homer's Odyssey*, Odysseus appointed Mentor as advisor to the young Telemachus. The dictionary defines 'mentor' as 'experienced and trusted advisor'. The use of mentors has become fairly widespread throughout the NHS over recent years. The term started to appear in management literature in the 1970s.

Mentors are individuals who enter into a special working relationship with another person, usually a more junior colleague, to act as their advisor, counsellor and even role model.

It often involves a senior keeping an interest in the development of a protegé through a significant aspect of his or her career. Mentors may be asked to adopt a high-flier on a course or provide advice or assistance to a young professional. The role may be informal, where a senior takes an active interest in the career development of a trainee, and could also be regarded as developing a support network. The core capabilities have been identified as self-awareness (under-standing self); behavioural awareness (understanding others); professional insight; sense of proportion and good humour; communication competence; conceptual modelling; commitment to own continued learning; a strong interest in developing others; building and maintaining relationships; and goal clarity (Clutterbuck 2000).

Mentoring demands a close professional relationship between individuals. It involves a long-term supportive relationship involving assessment, career guidance and often counselling. Mentors need a wide range of assessment, appraisal and counselling skills. Mentors are usually more senior individuals, chosen for their perceived wisdom by the learner, but can also be peers in a group.

Counselling

Doctors, often without extensive psychological training, are from time to time called on to deal with troubled people, sometimes patients and sometimes colleagues. Although not professional counsellors, they are often regarded as well suited (or the nearest available) to address the woes of others.

The aim of a one-to-one interaction may be to solve a serious personal problem faced by someone who has brought it to you on the assumption that you will be able to help. Common sense demands that, if you judge the problem to be beyond your capability, you should direct the person to someone more suited to advise them. Frequently, however, it may be within your power to help someone resolve their problem by merely acting as a sounding board. This does not, however, involve playing a passive role.

The aims of such counselling may include:

• clarifying problem issues
• facilitating problem solving
• encouraging insight.

It will *not* include:

• curing mental health problems
• relieving drug or alcohol dependency
• removing all suffering
• solving social or political problems.

Common factors in an effective approach will usually involve:

- listening
- encouraging
- exploring
- following the lead given by the client.

The most critical of these is listening, which is covered in detail below.

Personal counselling

The contents of personal counselling are confidential. They generally deal with personal, social, family, cultural or spiritual issues which are affecting performance at work or life generally. It should only be carried out when explicitly agreed by the individuals concerned.

Carrying out personal counselling requires training in counselling skills. Thus counselling should only be carried out within the limits of the individual's training, and they should recognise when to refer on to a more experienced or more highly trained counsellor. Nevertheless, basic level counselling can be a valuable attribute of many doctors who interact with trainees.

Counselling is non-judgemental, except when the law is broken. Personal counselling may lead to a referral to psychiatric help or individual, group or family therapy.

Career counselling

Career counselling uses methods to assess attitudes, values, personal attributes, skills and knowledge to inform a career choice. This may be necessary for doctors (and medical students) at or before crossroads in their careers. Career counselling requires the counsellor to have counselling skills, a wide range of knowledge of medical careers and ready access to career information and the consequences of each choice. There is a danger of career counselling developing into persuasion followed by patronage, leading to unfairness and in potentially poor career choice.

Career guidance

Career guidance differs from career counselling in that the individual is advised about their chosen career pathway. Guidance usually requires someone to have a detailed knowledge of that particular career pathway and may include assessment of the stage of training reached.

Note: Career counselling and career guidance are sometimes confused and used interchangeably. It is important that it is clear whether the process is about making a career choice between a variety of careers or dealing with an already chosen career.

Effective listening

We spend half our working lives in situations in which we are supposed to be listening. For most of this time we are doing anything but listening. We might be hearing what is being said, but our minds are often distracted by other thoughts and our behaviour sends signals to the other person indicating this fact. Effective (or active) listening is a developed skill and one worth acquiring. Effective listening benefits include:

- gaining a better understanding of what people feel and what is happening
- improved working relationships
- reduced conflict
- new ideas and perspectives on issues.

Guidelines for effective listening
- Prepare yourself to listen by putting your own ideas on hold while you concentrate.
- Avoid distractions from visitors, interruptions, telephone calls, the window etc.
- Listen to the whole message – content, tone and non-verbal cues.
- Be silent, attentive and interested.
- Be receptive and keep an open mind.
- Allow the speaker to finish.
- Take notes where appropriate.
- Respect confidences and build trust.
- Clarify and summarise.
- Reflect feelings to encourage the speaker to be open.

Giving feedback

If you ask people to reflect on some of the more significant aspects of their personal development they will often talk about people who have given them direct and pertinent information about themselves. This personal help can be useful but sometimes people are hurt by the feedback they receive. So we need to explore ways of giving feedback which enable the person to be stronger as a result. These guidelines may help you give and receive feedback in the most constructive way.

You may have to work at it to be effective but the skills developed will not only be a valuable management asset but can influence and improve your own personal life.

Poorly performing colleagues

Recognition that a colleague is performing below an acceptable professional standard brings with it a heavy responsibility. Patients and other colleagues depend on the professionalism of all those around them. There are conflicting loyalties, however, which can make the decision to address this type of problem a difficult one. The key is often in identifying the problem early. The three most common causes of poor performance in colleagues are alcoholism, drug abuse and clinical depression. They all share a slow onset and lack of insight into one's problem. This insidious process may also make it difficult to decide when a sick colleague needs help. With hindsight, it can often be easy to spot the onset. There is also the reasonable concern that if allegations are found to be groundless, you could be vulnerable to litigation in slander or libel and end up before a civil court or the GMC. This is said to be very rare, however.

Establishing facts is vital before taking action. Unfortunately this is not always easy. As in so many cases it is the 'evidence' and its quality or provability that is crucial. For example, smelling alcohol on the breath of a poorly performing colleague early in the morning is difficult to prove. But if a number of people have done so on a number of occasions and are prepared to sign and date statements, then that is better evidence.

The GMC has published a booklet on *Good Medical Practice* which stresses your duty to protect patients if you believe a colleague's performance or health is a threat. Before taking any action you need to ascertain the facts and it is often helpful, and certainly sensible, to discuss your concerns with an experienced colleague before notifying the employing authority on regulatory body.

The Central Consultants and Specialists Committee (CCSC) has also produced guidance on the actions that consultants should take if they are concerned about the performance of colleagues. They highlight the following:

- act quickly to protect patients
- places clear professional responsibility to take action where there are serious concerns
- the first step may be to discuss with senior colleague or colleague in specialty from another hospital
- consider the use of local informal procedures (e.g. 'Three Wise Men' or equivalent)
- possibly seek advice from the local BMA office
- it may be necessary to bring the matter to the attention of your trust through the medical director, clinical director or even the chief executive.

There are a number of agencies available to help doctors in these situations:

- GMC's Fitness to Practice Directorate (Tel: 0207 580 7642). The switchboard will put you through for informal advice about GMC regulations.
- The BMA 24–hour stress counselling service for doctors (Tel: 0645 200169).
- The British Doctors' and Dentists' Group, via Medical Council on Alcoholism (Tel: 0207 487 4445)
  A Support group of medical and dental drug and alcohol abusers.
- The Association of Anaesthetists' Sick Doctor Scheme (Tel: 0207 631 1650)
  For all anaesthetists, including those in training. The telephone number is a main switchboard that will channel you through to an appropriate person.
- Doctors' Support Network (Tel: 07071 223372)
  Self-help group.
- The Sick Doctor's Trust (Tel: 01252 345163)
- Counsel for Sick Doctors (Tel: 0207 935 5982)

Key learning points

Preparation – teaching and appraisal are each made more effective if both trainer *and* trainee come prepared.

Agenda – appraisal meetings should follow an agenda which should be agreed before or at the start of the meeting.

Giving feedback – negative feedback is made more acceptable if it is preceded by positive remarks about the appraisee. Even better, get them to tell you about the weaker areas of their performance.

Setting objectives – all objectives should meet the criteria of being SMART.

Dealing with conflict – if conflict is not easily resolved, the trainee should be transferred to the responsibility of another trainer.

Managing the confidentiality issue – confidentiality can be crucial in getting the appraisee to open up about weaknesses, but it has to be made clear that behaviour which contravenes GMC or other regulations will lead to disclosure to others.

Avoid taking on trainee's problems – these may be simply to do with training activities. The trainee should carry some responsibility for organising their own learning. Additionally, you should recognise that your role as an appraiser does not make you an expert counsellor. If serious problems are disclosed, refer them to someone who is equipped to help them.

Related reading

Bulstrode C and Hunt V (1996) *Educating Consultants*. Oxford University Press, Oxford.

Clutterbuck D (1985) *Everyone Needs a Mentor*. IPM, London.

Clutterbuck D (2000) 'Ten core mentor competencies'. Organisations and people. *AMED*. 7(4): 29–34.

Gatrell J and White T (2000) *Medical Appraisal, Selection and Revalidation*. RSM Press, London.

General Medical Council (1997) *The New Doctor*. GMC, London

Marteau TM, Wynne G, Kaye W and Evans TR (1990) Resuscitation: experience without feedback increases confidence but not skill. *BMJ*. **300**: 849–50.

NHSE (1998) *A Guide to Specialist Registrar Training* (The Orange Book). DoH, London.

Prior J (1994) *Handbook of Training and Development* (2e). Gower/ITD, Aldershot.

RCS (1996) *Training the Trainers*. Raven Department of Education, The Royal College of Surgeons of England, London.

Singer EJ (1974) *Effective Management Coaching*. IPM, London.

The Standing Committee on Postgraduate Medical and Dental Education (1996) *Appraising Doctors and Dentists in Training: a working paper for consultation*. SCOPME, London.

6

Clinical governance, quality and research

This chapter aims to develop understanding of the role of clinical governance in delivering a quality healthcare service. It explores the role of risk management, clinical audit and research. It also describes current developments in NHS structures and initiatives for improving quality of service.

Introduction

Past quality-related initiatives in the NHS have been at best fragmented. Current attempts to improve quality systems in the NHS seek to produce clear evidence-based guidelines, place responsibility for quality of local care on trust boards and professional and managerial staff, and ensure that the process is adequately monitored. Clinical governance was introduced in the context of these aims.

Some years after its introduction there is still considerable confusion over the meaning of the term 'clinical governance' and, more especially, how it should be implemented. It is concerned with assuring clinical quality, and encompasses themes of risk management and professional accountability. Quality is elusive both as a concept and in day-to-day working but there is constant pressure to improve it. This is partly due to the inherent complexity of healthcare and the fact that patients and their families often have only partial insight into what constitutes good or bad treatment. So there is a reliance on professionals for what is called an 'agency relationship'. There is continuing debate about the ability of professionals to self-govern, particularly as the media and public have been concerned by the current structures. Earlier attempts to overcome some of these concerns included the introduction of medical and clinical audit in the early 1990s.

Quality comes in different forms. Quality assurance is making sure not only that the right things get done, but also that the wrong things do not. In clinical practice, audit has been described as a shield of quality. Mistakes matter and, some believe, will always happen. By finding good criteria to work to and sticking to them we can make dramatic improvements in performance.

In this chapter we will cover a number of issues that are linked to quality. According to the Chief Medical Officer (1998) the pursuit of quality can be broken down into three distinct but interrelated strands:

• clinical governance
• enhanced professional self-regulation
• lifelong learning.

Medical research can contribute to improved patient care and involvement in research can be a powerful aid to learning and understanding. It can also contribute to career development. The research process is also covered in this chapter.

In the 1950s and 1960s it was often assumed that more spending on healthcare would lead to better health. Increased awareness of other determinants of health, such as housing, employment, family and social class positioning, has induced a more political approach. Other factors such as the oil crisis of the 1970s, the emergence of previously non-industrial countries as strong economic competitors, the increasing cost of new health technologies and the growing proportion of the aged population, have led to increased pressure to contain costs. The creation of the NHS internal market as part of the reforms in the late 1980s and early 1990s was accompanied by a plethora of initiatives aimed at improving quality. More recently quality has become focused on evidence-based medicine. In clinical practice one could regard audit as a requirement of quality control. First let us consider some of the main issues around quality in healthcare.

What does quality mean in a health service?

Although it is suggested that quality improvements will save money, there are two questions regarding improvement in care:

• related to the service – is it in some way superior to others?
• related to the patient – did it speed recovery; was it comfortable and painless?

There are always at least two points of view, the doctor's and the patient's. Does the definition lie in the relationship between the two points of view? The service may be excellent but it is not important unless valued by the patient. The delivery process also has to be excellent. The relationship is difficult in the health service where expectations and requirements of many parties in the system may be very different. The following are some established definitions of quality:

• fitness for purpose (Juran 1986)

- conformance to requirements (Crosby 1984)
- the totality of features and characteristics of a product or service that bear on its ability to satisfy stated or implied needs (ISO8402 1986)
- the degree of conformance of all the relevant features and characteristics of the product (or service) to all aspects of a customer's need, limited by the price and delivery he or she will accept (Groocock 1986).

These are all about meeting a customer's need, or alternatively cannot be improved by adding something they do not need, nor achieved if wanted now but not available until later. For the NHS, the suggested definition is:

- quality service meets all the requirements of customers, stated or implied, while keeping costs at a minimum.

The word 'customer' may feel uncomfortable, but we have a range of customers with different requirements. These include patients, their relatives, general practitioners, other staff within the hospital, providers, purchasers and the general public. Perhaps the word 'stakeholder' fits better in this context.

Accepting that there are some differences between health and other industries, various authors have tried to define quality in health. Maxwell (1984) identified six dimensions:

- access to services
- equity
- relevance to need
- social acceptability
- efficiency
- effectiveness.

Working for Patients (1989) produced a set of seven factors focused more on patients:

- appropriateness of treatment and care
- achievement of optimum clinical outcome
- clinically recognised procedures to minimise complications and similar preventable events
- attitude which treats patients with dignity and as individuals
- environment conducive to patient safety, reassurance and contentment
- speed of response to patient needs and minimum inconvenience to them (and their relatives and friends)
- involvement of patients in their own care.

Stevens, Colin-Jones and Gabbay (1995) usefully draw together themes in making decisions about interventions and quality. Their paper is well worth reading as it provides guidance for ordering one's thoughts and also introduces Buxton's Law: 'it is always too early to evaluate a new technology until, unfortunately, suddenly it's too late'. It sets out seven stages needed for assessing technology (loaded towards new technology, but highly applicable to existing technologies) and emphasises the importance of both analysis – drawing together information from a wide range of sources to bolster evidence from systematic review and meta-analysis – and costs, which have to be dealt with pragmatically.

The article is a good, basic guide to making decisions based on levels of evidence and cost per QALY (quality-adjusted life year) and in a recent review Bandolier (1999) remarked: 'Pragmatism is the name of the game . . . It is worth having a copy of this thoughtful and influential paper on your desk for re-reading at quiet moments'.

Quality management

What is quality management? The subject is surrounded by jargon, buzzwords and phrases. These include quality control, quality assurance, total quality management (TQM), zero defects, continuous quality improvement (CQI) among many others. Are they relevant to healthcare? Why all this fuss about quality? The answer lies in changes in attitudes and expectations in the community. There is now more information about how well services perform. People are increasingly encouraged to expect higher standards and quality in goods and services. But 'how?' has been the concern of many in health services. According to the internationally known quality guru Deming (1986), 'Management is responsible for 94% of quality problems and their first step should be to dismantle the barriers that prevent employees doing a good job'. Government responded to the perceived need for improved quality by publishing *The Patient's Charter* in 1991. The World Health Organization (1983) defined quality assurance in healthcare in one sentence of over 110 words!

Implementing quality improvements is a major task requiring the commitment of all involved in the delivery of service. Measuring patient satisfaction, while essential, is not the only dimension of quality of care. Professionals have the principal responsibility for defining and maintaining technical standards (Richards 1986). Quality has to be built in to the system – failures cannot be thrown away!

Total quality management (TQM)

This term is frequently used to describe an organisational approach to quality improvement. The requirements of TQM are said to be:

- commitment and example from top management
- an organisation-wide commitment to quality

- an approach which focuses on the customer (patient)
- a participative environment and teamwork
- pursuit of continuous improvement
- quality of suppliers.

One of the clearest approaches to implementing a quality policy is that described by Crosby (1984) through the notion of 'zero defects'. This addresses some of the issues in which this might be relevant to healthcare, with a case study in general practice. It also addresses the question 'can we afford *(not)* to improve quality?'. It addresses the four main cost elements:

- costs of prevention
- costs of appraisal
- internal failure costs
- external failure costs.

Benchmarking

Another frequently used term, defined by the UK Benchmarking Centre (1993) as the continuous, systematic search for best practices, and for the implementation process which will lead to superior performance.

Purpose:

- helps you understand how you compare with other organisations
- promotes understanding of the performance 'gap' between organisations
- assists in the search to find and implement best practice
- helps to identify areas for process improvement.

Relevance to the NHS:

- demonstrates value for resources in a resource-constrained environment with increasing service user expectations
- offers measure of outcomes
- defines targets for effectiveness
- offers the opportunity to share value for money improvements both within sites and between other parts of the NHS.

Evidence-based medicine (EBM) and evidence-based healthcare (EBH)

Evidence-based medicine and healthcare are essentially about quality. Quality in trying to find studies that address a question, ensuring that only unbiased studies are included, and distilling that information. Of course there is another quality when the knowledge is combined with a doctor's education and experience and knowledge of a patient to make sensible decisions. EBH has been defined as 'the conscientious, explicit and judicious use of current best evidence in making decisions about the care of individual patients' (Sackett *et al.* 1996). It is the opposite of conjecture-based decision making. Many organisations, journals and electronic databases are dedicated to its pursuit and encouraging its growth in the NHS. This growth will undoubtedly continue, given financial pressures and the requirements of clinical governance.

The problem may sometimes be an over-abundance of evidence, which is in academic format and widely dispersed. EBH information is increasingly available electronically and the following is a list of some of the sources.

Medline Bibliographic citations and author abstracts from around 3900 current international biomedical journals. Nine million records dating back to 1966. It is the chief database of the US National Library of Medicine.

Cochrane Library Published quarterly on CD-ROM. Part of the Cochrane Centre, itself part of the EBH network known as The Cochrane Collaboration. The NHS Centre for Reviews and Dissemination is a sibling organisation based at York University – it can be accessed at www.york.ac.uk/inst/crd.centre.htm.

Bandolier A monthly journal produced for the NHS Research and Development Directorate. It provides surveys, evaluation and comments on a wide range of conditions and treatments. See www.jr2.ox.ac.uk/bandolier.

Ovid's Evidenced Based Medicine Reviews This database pools EBH literature references from the Cochrane database and *Best Evidence*, a database containing US effectiveness literature. See www.ovid.com/product/ebmr/ebmr.htm.

Centre for Evidence Based Medicine Provides EBM resources.
See www.cebm.jr2.ox.ac.uk.

Centre for Evidence Based Dentistry Encourages clinical enquiry and debate among dentists. See www.ihs.ox.ac.uk.

Centre for Evidence Based Child Health Run by the Institute for Child Health at Great Ormond Street Hospital for Children, London.
See www.ich.bpmf.ac.uk/ebm/centre.

Institute for Public Health, University of Cambridge Evaluates interventions and preventive medicine in primary and secondary care. See www.iph.cam.ac.uk.

Centre for Evidence Based Mental Health   Provides information related to EBH in mental health. See www.psychiatry.ox.ac.uk/cebmh.html.

NHS quality initiatives

The New NHS White Paper (1997) insisted there would be no rationing in the new NHS. Priorities are to be set in a variety of ways and by a variety of bodies, with the underlying principle that only treatments proven to be cost-effective are allowed. The government tries to help trusts cost their services by publishing a National Schedule of Reference Costs (NSRC).

Improving quality is stated to be at the heart of *The New NHS*, which sets out several ways to try and achieve better standards. The following organisations and initiatives exist to contribute to the maintenance and improvement of quality in healthcare. Some have already been referred to, but to remind you . . .

Clinical governance

All trusts are legally required to ensure they implement systems that ensure the provision of quality services. To achieve this they must implement 'clinical governance' (*see* p. 154).

Commission for Health Improvement (CHI)

Established in 1999, CHI was established to 'monitor, assure and improve clinical quality'. Its members include healthcare professionals, managers, academics and patient representatives. If it uncovers serious or persistent problems it will 'work with the organisation on lasting remedies'. CHI is not concerned with issues covered by the General Medical Council nor the principle of professional self-regulation. It promotes excellence by identifying and addressing local quality problems through visits and spot checks. NHS regional offices and health authorities are responsible for ensuring that its recommendations are enforced. It reports on progress annually to the Secretary of State for Health.

National Institute for Clinical Excellence (NICE)

Set up in March 1999, NICE is made up of a board of healthcare professionals, managers, academics, economists and patient representatives to work on and produce clinical guidelines. The aim is 'to ensure that best practice is shared and spread across the country'. It is a special health authority that produces formal advice for clinicians and managers on the clinical- and cost-effectiveness of new and existing technologies, including medicines, diagnostic tests and surgical procedures.

It has a six-stage approach:

- to identify new health interventions or examine current practice
- to undertake research to collect evidence
- to consider the evidence on clinical- and cost-effectiveness and produce guidance
- to disseminate guidance
- to implement at local level through clinical governance and other approaches
- to monitor the impact and keep advice under review.

It is expected to produce about 10–15 scientifically-based guidelines each year. See www.nice.org.uk.

Health Improvement Programmes (HImP)

HImPs are 'the local strategy for improving health and healthcare', drawn up by health authorities in consultation with trusts, PCGs and other primary care professionals and patients. Local authorities also have an input. They began in 1999 and are updated annually. PCGs ensure that the services they provide and commission are in tune with the priorities set out in the HImP.

National Service Frameworks (NSFs)

The NHSE works with the professions to draw up consistent nationwide quality standards as to what patients with specific diseases can expect to receive in the NHS. These are then incorporated into service agreements. They are issued by the Department of Health in conjunction with NICE and specify the type of service that should be available in all primary care, local hospital and specialist centres. CHI will ensure that these standards are met locally. Health authorities implement the standards of NSFs as part of the HImPs.

Critical Appraisal Skills Programme (CASP)

CASP was set up in 1993 by the NHSE and Anglia and Oxford Region to help healthcare professionals develop skills to evaluate evidence about the effectiveness of clinical products and treatments. It has grown in response to demand. It stages workshops and produces learning resources such as an interactive CD-ROM. See http://fester.his.path.cam.ac.uk/phealth/casphome.htm.

NHS Economic Evaluation Database

Based at York University's Centre for Reviews and Dissemination, the database contains abstracts of healthcare economic evaluations from various sources, bibliographic references to cost studies, papers on economic evaluations methodology and reviews of economic evaluations. See www.york.ac.uk/inst/crd/info.htm.

Accreditation and inspection programmes

Hospitals and other health facilities may have their organisation, management and clinical practices evaluated by an external body – a process known as accreditation. This leads to recognition that a service has achieved certain standards.

An important part of the process is initial self-assessment prior to inspection by outside assessors to assess the standards required. Following inspection, assessors submit a report that might indicate areas for improvement. Accreditation is for a fixed term and may also be applied in the context of recognition of a training programme.

Clinical guidelines

Clinical guidelines or protocols often set out treatment pathways and suggest options. An important function is to stop the use of established but unduly hazardous treatments, as well as discouraging the use of ineffective and possibly expensive treatments. They have become a component of clinical governance. NICE has a central role in co-ordinating work on guidelines.

National Centre for Clinical Audit (NCCA)

The NCCA was set up in 1995 to promote the use of clinical audit and to disseminate useful information.

NHS Beacon Services

The Department of Health has set aside £10m to fund beacon services (individual examples of best practice) and to help those conferred with beacon status spread improvement by organising open days, secondments and seminars as well as using the NHSnet to pass on information. Some of the funding also goes to trusts and practices who want to start applying the lessons learned from beacon sites. The best in each region will gain recognition through the annual Nye Bevan Award.

National Confidential Enquiries

These have been established over a number of years to examine clinical performance and serious avoidable events. The first began in 1951 examining the death of women during childbirth. The results of each enquiry are expected to feed into guidance and standards produced by NICE. In 1998, participation became compulsory.

The four areas of enquiries are:

- the National Confidential Enquiry into Perioperative Deaths (NCEPOD)
- the Confidential Enquiry into Stillbirths and Deaths in Infancy (CESDI)
- the Confidential Enquiry into Maternal Deaths (CEMD)
- the Confidential Enquiry into Suicide and Homicide by people with mental illness (CISH).

The GMC's *Maintaining Good Medical Practice Guide*

This is a booklet published by the GMC designed to strengthen the process of professional self-regulation. It provides advice on how to maintain good practice, what to do in cases of poor practice, the procedures involved and whom to contact.

Action on clinical audit

This is a two-year project set up in 1998 and funded by the NHSE to improve clinical audit in 22 NHS trusts. It investigates how clinical practice can be changed through audit.

Clinical Practice Evaluation Programme (CPEP)

This is part of the RCGP's quality initiative designed to help GPs across the UK evaluate and compare their care with equivalent practices.

Clinical Standards Board (Scotland) (CSBS)

This was set up in 1999 to act as the Scottish equivalent of the CHI in England. It links up with Scotland's Clinical Effectiveness Group and liases with NICE although its role is not to assess the cost-effectiveness of drugs. Its priority areas are cancer, coronary heart disease and mental health.

Continuing medical education (CME) and continuing professional development (CPD)

Lifelong learning and continuing education are a stated part of the NHS Human Resources Agenda. This states that NHS organisations must provide programmes on education and training, and personal and organisational development particularly around clinical governance. CME and CPD support healthcare professionals. There is, for example, a network of postgraduate medical centres based at district general hospitals. The medical Royal Colleges regard the encouragement of CPD as one of their key responsibilities.

National Framework for Assessing Performance (NFAP)

This framework was established in 1989/9 to broaden the definition of efficiency in the NHS. It collates a range of information to provide a meaningful assessment of performance and provides the basis for the NHS league tables.

It aims to cover areas of fair access, effectiveness of delivery of appropriate healthcare, patient or carer experiences, health outcomes of NHS care and the extent to which the NHS provides an efficient service. *See also* the section on IT in Chapter 3, p. 87.

Clinical governance

The market-oriented approach to healthcare raised concerns that the NHS had become too focused on financial and productivity issues. At the same time there had been a number of serious failings in clinical care that were given a lot of news coverage. The response of the Labour government was to publish *The New NHS: modern, dependable* White Paper in 1997, which set out how the internal market was to be replaced by 'a more integrated system of care with quality at its core'. There were equivalent Scottish and Welsh White Papers, *Designed to Care* and *Putting Patients First.* These set up a new structure to determine clinical and service standards, and monitor and compare performance against explicit targets. The White Paper started with the premise that trusts had been giving undue emphasis to the achievement of financial targets to the detriment of service quality. By giving trust boards the statutory duty to manage quality as well as their continuing financial duties, it sought to align clinical quality and financial responsibility. The internal market was blamed for fragmentation, unfairness, distortion, inefficiency, bureaucracy, instability and secrecy. There were renewed attempts to raise quality, increase efficiency and improve performance.

A subsequent consultation document *A First Class Service: quality in the new NHS* (1998) addressed quality in more detail. In the context of clinical governance, its recommendations included setting up:

• National Service Frameworks
• the Commission for Health Improvement (CHI)
• the National Framework for Assessing Performance
• the National Survey of Patient and User Experience.

At local level, PCG/Ts are expected to promote quality through service agreements that specify quality standards. Primary care also has to maintain a clinical governance framework.

Clinical governance links the elements. The reforms of 1997/8 resulted in the formation of the EQUIP Group at the Department of Health to implement quality. Chaired by the Chief Medical Officer (CMO) and Chief Nursing Officer (CNO) this group took a leading role in establishing clinical governance. Clinical governance imposes a statutory requirement on trusts to implement local systems for the assurance of quality of care; and this extends the existing system of professional self-regulation to local level.

The New NHS White Paper added a new duty of quality on trusts and primary care providers in addition to their financial duties. The government wanted clinicians to continue to be involved in management and in particular to take a lead in developing quality in clinical services, and coined the phrase 'clinical governance' to describe this. It recognised that provider chief executives are as accountable for quality as for finances, and that doctors' roles in management are now a necessity, no longer just an aspiration. Clinical governance committees of clinicians should be set up to facilitate this. They will cover audit, risk management, adverse event reporting and actions arising, and complaints management. Clinical directorates should submit regular quality reports to the trust board.

Ask any group of doctors or managers to complete the sentence 'Clinical governance is . . .' and you will almost certainly receive many different answers, all probably relevant. This suggests that clinical governance cannot be explained in a single term. Our research suggests that the term originated from two sources. First, corporate governance, a process outside healthcare which was described by Cadbury (1992) and Nolan (1995) as a basis for controls assurance in enterprise and public life. Second, it was based on the premise that managers and clinicians had not sufficiently engaged in quality initiatives and should be encouraged to embrace this new approach.

Professor Liam Donaldson is usually cited as the originator of the term (Scally and Donaldson 1998). Clinical governance is a mix of existing clinical risk management and quality procedures. It includes action to ensure that risks are avoided; adverse events are rapidly detected, openly investigated and lessons are learned from them; good practice is rapidly disseminated; and systems are in place to ensure continuous improvement in clinical care. The White Paper calls this a 'quality organisation'.

For an original definition of clinical governance you need to return to the 1997 White Paper, *The New NHS*, in which the fundamental principle placed the assurance of clinical quality at the same level as the financial wellbeing of healthcare organisations. Clinical governance was an attempt to provide mechanisms to monitor the quality of clinical practice. This was intended to lead to a fundamental change in attitude and culture within the NHS.

The government's consultation document *Clinical Governance: quality in the new NHS* (1999) defines it as 'A framework through which NHS organisations are accountable for continuously improving the quality of their services and safeguarding high standards of care by creating an environment in which excellence in clinical care will flourish.' A more succinct definition might be 'corporate responsibility for clinical quality'.

Continuing professional development is a central component. It brings together many of the areas covered in this chapter and Figure 6.1 tries to capture this. It sets out the areas at three levels – the setting of standards, the delivery of those standards and the monitoring process.

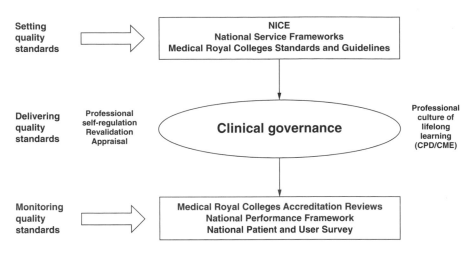

Figure 6.1 Factors critical to clinical governance.

Implementing clinical governance

The following systems and mechanisms contribute to clinical governance:

- clinical audit
- risk management
- health needs assessment
- evidence-based clinical practice
- patient feedback
- continuing professional development
- accreditation of healthcare providers
- development of clinical leadership skills
- effective management of poorly performing colleagues
- systems to ensure critical incidents are openly investigated and lessons learned are implemented.

The introduction of clinical governance has implications for individuals and organisations, and requires healthcare organisations to:

- develop leadership skills among clinicians (*see* Chapter 2)
- develop mechanisms to ensure that change in clinical practice occurs as a result of audit, risk management and complaints findings, thus closing the 'audit loop'
- develop appropriate accountability structures
- work more collaboratively and effectively between primary and secondary care
- develop more effective multi-disciplinary working

- build continuing medical education and continuing professional development into quality improvement programmes
- improve the information infrastructure of the NHS.

Trust chief executives are ultimately responsible to their boards for assuring the quality of services provided. Trust boards frequently set up clinical governance sub-committees, chaired by a clinical professional. A reporting regime requires trust boards to receive monthly quality reports and publish annual quality statements. At directorate level, a clinician supported by management ensures systems are in place for implementing clinical governance. Models in individual trusts do vary.

Actions

Check the following are in place in your trust.

- Quality improvement programmes (e.g. clinical audit).

- Leadership skills are developed at clinical team level.

- Evidence-based practice is in day-to-day use.

- Evaluated good practice and innovation are disseminated within and outside the organisation.

- Clinical risk reduction programmes.

- Adverse events are detected, openly investigated and the lessons learned applied.

- Lessons for clinical practice are learned from complaints made by patients.

- Problems of poor clinical performance are recognised early and dealt with to prevent harm to patients.

- All professional development programmes reflect the principles of clinical governance.

- Quality of data collected to monitor clinical care is itself of a high standard.

Risk management

Risk management adopts a formal and systematic process to identify and analyse risk and take remedial action to reduce or eliminate the risk of harm to patients, staff and the organisation. Both *The New NHS* (1997) and *Clinical Governance: quality in the new NHS* (1999) placed clinical risk management as a key component of clinical governance. They required clear policies to be implemented which were aimed at managing risk and supporting professional staff in identifying and tackling poor performance. The stated aim was to protect patients and NHS resources. Critical incident reporting systems should ensure that events are openly investigated and lessons learned and quickly applied. Similar action should be taken to ensure complaints procedures are fair to patients, their families and staff. Staff should be supported in reporting their concerns so that early action can be taken to remedy a situation before patients are harmed.

There is always a measure of risk associated with healthcare interventions. The MDU (1999) reported a 1991 Harvard study that examined over 30 000 records randomly selected from 51 hospitals in New York State. An adverse events incidence of nearly 4% was uncovered, many of which they concluded were due to negligence and contributed to prolonged disability or even death. There are similar studies from other countries. Poor quality or ill-informed advice can cause harm and seriously undermine patient confidence in the service provided.

Three major studies of adverse incidents in clinical practice revealed important findings (Mills 1977; Brennan *et al.* 1991 and Leape *et al.* 1991; Wilson *et al.* 1995). These all used two stages. First, medical records were screened retrospectively against criteria designed to identify potential adverse risk. Then a clinician/lawyer panel conducted an in-depth review of those identified cases to see whether the patient suffered any adverse event. The three studies showed adverse event rates of 4.65%, 3.7% and 16.6% respectively.

An adverse event is defined as an unintended injury caused by clinical intervention, as distinct from the disease process, which is sufficiently serious to lead to temporary or permanent impairment or disability in the patient.

How can risks be identified?

Various sources and methods are used to identify risks. These might include any or all of the following:

- critical incident reporting
- clinical audits
- complaints procedures

- confidential enquiry findings
- observations of staff
- reports by investigative committees
- accreditation visit reports
- patient satisfaction surveys.

Systems embedded in the working of healthcare organisations are seen as the only means of ensuring continuing responsiveness to risk management needs. The alternative is a 'crisis management' approach, dealing with problems as they arise, which adds risk and cost.

Clinical audit

Audit is a contractual requirement for doctors in hospital and community services. GPs are not mandated through their contracts, although the demands of clinical governance make it essential that they undertake audit to meet professional requirements. GPs are required to report to their PCG/T on the process and outcomes of audits undertaken by them. There is, therefore, an expectation that all healthcare professionals would participate in audit. However, a culture has developed that makes it difficult for audit to excite many doctors. Nevertheless, audit is closely related to education, evidence-based medicine, research and quality. A commonly asked question at medical interviews is 'What is the difference between audit and research?' or, less often, 'Describe the link between audit and education'. Some suggestions for answers are given below.

Audit derives from the Latin 'to hear'. *The Oxford Dictionary* defines it as 'official examination of accounts'. Clinical audit is 'the systematic, critical analysis of the quality of clinical care'. Participation in clinical audit was made mandatory for hospital doctors in the NHS reforms launched in 1989 and endorsed by the Royal Colleges, although it was voluntary for those in primary care and for other healthcare professionals.

Audit activity is generally high and in 1993 the Department of Health encouraged the development of multi-professional audit. It was seen as part of the educational process, forming part of clinical practice, based on the setting of standards with the potential to improve outcomes. It required managers to become involved in both the process and outcome, was confidential to both practitioner and patient, and involved patient input into the process.

Certain key principles were stated:

- maintaining and enhancing continuing professional education and development
- collaborative audit programmes to enhance integration across professions

- making audit mainstream within the business of the hospital by incorporating it into the quality strategy and involving general managers at all levels
- crossing the primary/secondary care interface by involving all key professionals from disease prevention, health promotion to rehabilitation and continuing care, and involving the patient in the audit process.

The success and effectiveness of clinical audit remains variable and it is better established in well-managed supportive organisations with good communication systems. The resource commitment required to establish an effective clinical audit programme is substantial and demands long-term commitment and support from top management levels. Audit has shifted from being a centrally-driven priority of the Department of Health to a locally-driven activity. Clinical audit demands skills in teamwork, identifying problems, process analysis, data collection and management, problem solving and a change in management skills that are not a key part of any one professional's training in healthcare. Training and education in clinical audit need to be seen as essential for everyone taking part in audit activities. Doctors, who are required to maintain records of their clinical performance for their revalidation folders, are reliant on effective clinical audit systems.

Clinical audit and research

Some quoted differences.

- Research is often deductive and concerned with critical testing.
- Control groups and validating measures are more likely to be used in research than audit.
- Audit is often concerned with small-scale problems requiring local solutions.
- The scope of research is likely to be different and to reach a wider national/ international audience through publication of results in academic journals.
- Research can provide answers in areas that audit could not tackle and challenges the efficacy of a particular therapy.
- Research raises questions about purposes (and means of achieving them).
- Audit evaluates what exists and takes purposes for granted.
- Audit ascertains whether the inputs and processes achieve the outcome desired.
- Audit and research can feed into each other.
- Audit can give rise to research questions; if the outcomes of audit are not what was intended, research can ask why.

Perhaps the easiest to remember is that research is about finding the right thing to do, and audit is about ensuring you are doing the right thing right!

Clinical audit and education

Some issues and links to consider.

- Clinical audit is a professional development activity that highlights educational needs in terms of audit methods and data analysis.
- By generating new knowledge, clinical audit can also contribute to postgraduate and undergraduate curricula in the healthcare professions.
- Education providers can use the knowledge gained through clinical audit to adapt curricula to new requirements, while providing health professionals with advice on research methods.

Medical audit was defined in the 1989 White Paper as 'the systematic, critical analysis of the quality of medical care, including the procedures used for diagnosis and treatment, the use of resources and the resulting outcome and quality of life for the patient'. Audit was formally introduced into the NHS in 1989, endorsed by the Royal Colleges and supported by specific funding from the DoH. The last year of protected funding, 1993/94, saw a total budget of £41.9m in England. Government encouragement for audit in general practice commenced in 1990 with funding being made available to FHSAs to support Medical Audit Advisory Groups (MAAGs). The nursing and therapy professions were encouraged to develop audit by the DoH in 1991. Again, specific funding was provided to pump-prime this activity and for 1993/94 the budget for England was £8.2m.

Types of audit

There are various types and classifications of audit in healthcare.

Medical audit

This was the original type when first formally introduced and was described as the systematic critical analysis of the quality of medical care including the procedures used for diagnosis and treatment, the use of resources and the resulting outcome and quality of life for the patient.

Clinical audit

Clinical audit is like medical audit but involves all professionals, rather than just doctors.

Nursing audit

Methods which compare actual practice against pre-agreed guidelines and identify areas for improving their care. Examples include 'Monitor' and 'Qualpac'.

Prospective audit

Standards and measures are agreed at the start and are recorded for patients and their families during their care.

Retrospective audit

Looks back at the care of patients, usually by using medical records and extracting the information.

Multi-professional clinical audit

The move towards multi-professional clinical audit was encouraged by the DoH in 1993 as it was seen as an educational process, forming part of clinical practice and based on the setting of standards. It was also seen to generate results that could be used to improve outcomes, involve managers in both the process and outcome, be confidential at both patient and clinician level, and informed by the views of patients/clients.

Key principles that need to be built on in developing a multi-professional approach include:

- maintaining and enhancing the continuing education/professional development aspects
- the potential to enhance integration across professions by achieving collaborative audit programmes
- making audit mainstream business by integrating it within the corporate quality programme and involving general managers at all levels
- developing a plan that looks at the totality of healthcare from disease prevention and health promotion to treatment and rehabilitation
- working across the primary/secondary care interface involving the whole healthcare team
- emphasising the patient focus and input to the audit process.

Clinical audit cycle

Clinical audit is a cycle that follows a process of setting standards, collecting and analysing data, comparing these data to the standards in a peer-review process and then finally taking action to improve the quality of care. A vital part of the process is reflection on the service to reach agreement on the purpose and value of that service. This reflection has a two-fold role: first, helping the team to learn about each other's roles and second, ensuring they have jointly agreed what they are trying to achieve with their patients.

Another key element is the need to constantly evaluate clinical effectiveness in order to achieve health gain for patients. Factors to consider have been suggested by Batstone and Edwards (1994) as timeliness, appropriateness, process and effectiveness (TAPE).

Timeliness, appropriateness and effectiveness refer to the assessment of whether an intervention was the correct one, undertaken at the correct time and performed correctly. The process used by each individual professional in their contribution to the patient outcome is seen to need individual professional determination and judgement. So, for example, a nurse or physiotherapist is not judging whether a surgeon's technique is correct. In the same way it is inappropriate for a doctor to judge an occupational therapist's training skills.

For clinical audit to be successful it is important to focus all this activity at the healthcare team level. It is also important for audit to embrace questions of cost-effectiveness and value for money. Value for money is the best use of a finite resource, not cost-cutting.

Multi-professional audit must focus on patient issues rather than professional issues. With the growth of consumerism there is growing emphasis on lay input into the audit process, but the mechanisms for involving patients are not well developed. Focus groups have been used, particularly by mental health units. Another potential mechanism is to seek out users of the service and to train them to participate, but not to pick one or two 'professional' patients who may have their own agenda or pressure groups for the same reason.

The structure introduced to replace Community Health Councils is seen as giving a wider opportunity for lay persons to contribute directly to quality in the NHS.

Audit and professional development

We have already considered that one of the fundamental principles of clinical audit is that it is an educational process as well as being related to the moral and professional accountability for practice. Clinical audit can be seen as a means to develop the team by developing reflective practice.

Audit may also be linked to portfolio learning. Most of the medical Royal Colleges have developed systems of points for accreditation – these mainly relate to lectures and study days rather than experiential learning – but the potential for the learning that takes place through participation in the audit process can be recognised and accredited as part of any individual's continuing professional development. Records are maintained and kept in the revalidation folder as evidence of involvement in continuing professional development. These approaches are also in accord with the principles of adult learning and generate effective learning.

Audit demands skills in teamwork, identifying problems, process analysis, data collection and management, problem solving and a change in management skills that are not usually a key part of any one professional's training in healthcare. Thus training and education in clinical audit need to be seen as essential for everyone taking part in audit activities.

Implementing clinical audit

Key features of implementing clinical audit include:

- identifying significant problems
- analysing the circumstances and causes
- finding possible solutions through changes in practices, processes or organisational arrangements
- implementing solutions to produce lasting improvements in the quality of care.

A useful conceptual framework for implementing audit is to break it down into structure, process and outcomes.

Structure

Structure includes:

- resources used (i.e. equipment and human resources)
- training
- communication (e.g. a multi-disciplinary group and an individual professional group)
- patient trail or clinical activity studied
- quality indicators used
- agreed, achievable and measurable standards used for each above indicator
- specific outcomes
- action plan for improvement
- the action plan for ongoing audit
- answering the question 'How have we improved our service using audit?'.

Process

Process is about:

- negotiating or obtaining funds to carry out the audit

- acquiring the equipment required to carry out the audit, e.g. a computer
- recruiting assistance for collecting and analysing data
- setting up an appropriate group to advise on the way forward
- agreeing the main activity and providing the indicators to be agreed for each process
- agreeing standards with targets to be achieved and measured for each activity.

Outcome

Outcome is about:

- specifying measured outcomes
- creating an action plan for improvements
- demonstrating how services have been improved by using audit.

Action

Reflect on the credibility and quality of your audit experiences.

The organisation

- Is there a 'supra' trust group to co-ordinate audit?
- Is quality management and clinical audit combined or co-dependent?
- Is there central co-ordination of quality improvement initiatives?
- Are audit programmes scheduled far enough in advance to ensure participation by appropriate staff?
- Is there clear responsibility for the development and adoption of external and internal clinical guidelines?
- Are audit and quality management programmes incorporated in the business plan?

Resources

- Is there agreement on how much staff time should be allocated to audit and quality improvement?
- Are audit support staff accessible to all clinical staff in all directorates?
- Is there a mechanism to ensure they are appropriately used?
- Are aggregated data on diagnosis, procedures and diagnostic tests complete, accurate and available for clinical analysis?
- Do staff have access to information on standards, methods and results of relevant projects inside and outside the trust?
- Is there a training budget for audit and quality improvement?

Produce a brief report of a clinical audit you have been involved in and the changes which resulted. Present this to a small group of four or five participants who will review the report, listen to your presentation and evaluate the use of the models and their application.

Exercise

• Think of a suitable topic for your next departmental audit, perhaps discussing this with a colleague.

• Find out who is responsible for audit in your department.

• Find out how the audit programme of your department is reported. Is it to the clinical tutor perhaps?

• Obtain a copy of last year's departmental audit report and consider whether any of the findings have resulted in changes.

Research

Reliable, research-based information is fundamental to the successful implementation of clinical governance. Research findings need to be widely disseminated and doctors skilled in evaluating the data and information. Effective organisational communication systems and relevant information technology have an important part to play in the process.

This section provides general guidelines and insight into how to carry out research – it is not a tutorial on how to carry out research. Some suggestions for further reading are given at the end of the chapter. If you are considering undertaking research, you are strongly recommended to read the series of articles published in the *British Medical Journal* (1997) on a range of research-related issues.

'One of the characteristics of a profession is its ability to develop and validate a body of knowledge that is unique to itself' (Etzioni 1969). The delivery of patient care, the planning, organisation and management of the services, and the education of those who provide that care, should be firmly based on well-researched practice. On a more personal level, there are numerous reasons for doctors involving themselves in research. Knowledge and understanding are frequently founded in engagement with the discovery of new ways of working. Research is usually time consuming and expensive, so it is instructive to list reasons for your involvement – the following suggestions for undertaking research are based on Murrell *et al.* (1999).

The challenge: discovering something new and advancing the boundaries of scientific knowledge can create a great sense of achievement. It engages the imagination, the emotion and the intellect. In some ways it is like detective work, starting with a problem, charting the way through a process of investigation, building up the evidence, and moving towards conclusions that represent, perhaps, your unique way of interpreting the discovery.

Becoming a better doctor: research fosters characteristics such as logical thought, critical analysis and self-reliance. These are of substantial benefit in clinical practice and most doctors who have undertaken periods of research will probably agree that they are better doctors because of it. Research insight enables the interpretation and evaluation of research undertaken by others. It could be argued that all professional practice should be research based and research validated, providing not only patients with quality care and attention but also ensuring that those commissioning healthcare are getting value in the provision of the services.

Improving job prospects: higher, research-based qualifications and publications are of great value when applying for jobs. Not only do they represent an interest in improved patient care and scientific understanding, but also a desire to improve personal development.

Pursuing an academic career: research interests and publications in reputable refereed journals are essential if a career in academia is considered.

When to research

With sufficient time, research can be performed readily. Most doctors conduct research as part of an additional or higher degree, for example, an intercalated BSc, MSc, MD, MS/MCh, MPhil or PhD. The timeframe varies considerably and admission to such courses relates to clinical post, experience and interests. Particular attention must also be paid to funding and access to clinical posts upon completion of research.

Undertaking research

You are likely to be influenced by your planned area of specialisation, areas of special interest to you or questions already under study in the department in which you work. Interest and perceived importance of the topic are necessary in order to maintain motivation. You also need to ask yourself whether you can be unbiased in the chosen topic as there is little point in starting unless you are sure you can complete the project within the available time.

Literature review and theoretical context

A literature review is essential to ensure that your proposed research is new and has not been previously attempted. Successful techniques and results in similar studies are also useful in generating ideas and identifying methodologies to achieve the aims and objectives of the research. Internet searches are particularly valuable. Medline accesses bibliographic citations and author abstracts from around 3900 current international biomedical journals. It has nine million records dating back to 1966 and is the chief database of the US National Library of Medicine. It contains all the constituent journals in *Index Medicus* and DHSSDATA, which provides DHSS publications. DHSS, DoH and NHS publications and statistics and other data are also available on www.doh.gov.uk although some material is limited to users on NHSnet. DIALOG includes almost 400 different databases including Medline, which is also within Datastar. If you refer to the earlier section on evidence-based medicine and healthcare you will find other useful database sources (*see* p. 148). You can use the reference list for related papers to overcome much laborious searching and work through the best journals for your subject, scanning the contents lists for suitable papers.

Research framework

All good research needs a framework or a set of stages, not necessarily chronological, which should be systematically addressed whatever the scale of the project. The research process is best thought of as a cycle where, having worked through all the stages, you can find yourself back at the beginning, rethinking the topic and formulation of the study. Or you might get to the funding stage and then be obliged to lower your sights to a more modest undertaking because funding cannot be acquired. Each stage is interconnected with every other stage and may need to be considered accordingly. It is helpful, initially, to obtain an overview of the process by considering each stage independently.

1 Aims, objectives and hypotheses

Before beginning a study you should draw up a list of realistic aims and objectives or a working hypothesis to prove or disprove. The choice of methodological approach and/or study design must also be decided upon. Consideration must also be given to the timeframe for the study and the variable data forms (quantitative or qualitative).

In carrying out health research the range of possible methodologies is vast, stretching from classical experimental (scientific method) through a variety of structured and semi-structured designs including clinical trials and surveys, to ethnographic and qualitative approaches. A practical fact to consider is the resource implications of design choice, e.g. qualitative research is more often an individual activity relying on the skills of the researcher.

2 Resources, ethics, communications and access

You should be able to identify the resource implications of your study once you have reached the design stage, but do not forget the costs of travel in time and money. Do you need to seek approval from the local ethical committee for your research to go ahead? What steps are necessary to gain access to the subject group/ samples? Are there sufficient samples/subjects for a statistically significant result?

3 Construction of instruments and equipment

You will need to be working on the construction or selection of your study instruments such as forms for recording data, questionnaires, attitude scales or physical equipment (ethical committees may need to view those before approval is given). What are the disadvantages/advantages of these forms of equipment? Do more accurate methods exist? What techniques are used in similar studies?

4 Pilot study

A pilot study is essential to validate the experimental procedure before the study can continue to a logical conclusion. Experimental flaws in the design and collection of data can be identified and dealt with, preventing a waste of time and resources.

5 Data collection

Although data collection can be laborious it is essential and must be conducted on a scale sufficient to ensure statistical viability.

6 Data preparation and analysis

Ask yourself 'What analysis is required to test the research hypothesis? Are the data at the appropriate level of measurement for the planned statistical tests?'

7 Presentation of findings

Depending on the audience and reason for the research, different forms of presentation may be required. It is often necessary to present reasons for the research, current understanding of the area, methods, results and conclusions in a concise and understandable form so that people unfamiliar with the area will understand. Getting your research published for a wider audience, for example in a refereed medical journal, requires understanding, insight, judgement and patience. If you are new to this process, you are strongly advised to seek help from a more experienced researcher. Research journals provide guidelines for presentation. In addition, you should become fully familiar with the writing style of the target journal. *See* Chapter 3 for further guidance on writing a journal article.

8 Evaluation

A good evaluation should reflect on whether the research could be improved and how the results fit into the understanding of the subject as a whole. It is also an opportunity for considered speculation about the subject and how such research can be applied in a clinical setting.

9 Dissemination of findings

Research is pointless if the results and conclusions are not expressed to the relevant scientific/medical communities. Such dissemination of experience and information allows others to build upon completed research and apply the findings to the clinical setting. This can be achieved through talks, submission of research articles to appropriate journals (*see* Chapter 3) and the use of poster presentations.

Evaluating research undertaken by others

Evaluation of research must be balanced, trying to identify both strengths and weaknesses in the method and methodology. A purely negative fault-finding exercise can be counter productive. It should be done constructively, with the stages in the research process being used to build a sound argument for this purpose.

Ask yourself 'Was there ethical committee approval for questionnaires, attitude scales or physical equipment? Was there a pilot study and data collection to detect any flaws in the design? Were the methods of data collection and statistical analysis appropriate? Are the data at the appropriate level of measurement for the planned statistical tests? Was the presentation of the findings suitable? Does the discussion draw appropriate conclusions from the experimental results and realistically place them within current understanding of the subject? Were flaws and potential improvements discussed?'

It is often the role of those evaluating research to decide whether or not to make changes or innovations based on the findings and, although the researchers themselves make an enormous contribution to innovations and changes, they really only provide the stimulus for this process.

Related reading

Academic Medicine Group (1997) *Guidelines for Clinicians Entering Research.* Royal College of Physicians of London. London.

Albert T (2000) *Winning the Publications Game. how to write a scientific paper without neglecting your patients* (2e). Radcliffe Medical Press, Oxford.

Albert T (2000) *A–Z of Medical Writing.* British Medical Journal Books, London.

Bandolier (1999) **6**(2): 7.

Batstone GF (1990) Educational aspects of medical audit. *BMJ.* **301**: 326–8.

Batstone GF and Edwards M (1994) Clinical audit: how should we proceed? *Southampton Medical Journal.* **10**(1): 13–19.

Batstone GF and Edwards M (1996) Multi-professional audit. In: A White (ed) *Textbook of Management for Doctors.* Churchill Livingstone, Edinburgh.

Brennan TA, Leape LL, Laird NM *et al.* (1991) Incidence of adverse events and negligence in hospitalised patients. Results of Harvard Medical Practice Study I. *New England Journal of Medicine.* **324**: 370–6.

British Medical Journal series of articles (1997). *BMJ.* **315**.

Bowden D (1996) Risk management. In: A White (ed) *Textbook of Management for Doctors.* Churchill Livingstone, London.

Cadbury A (1992) *Report of the Committee on the Financial Aspects of Corporate Governance.* Gee and Co, London.

Chief Medical Officer (1998) *A Review of Continuing Professional Development in General Practice.* DoH, Leeds.

Department of Health (1998) *A First Class Service: quality in the new NHS.* DoH, London.

Dixon N (1991) *An Audit Primer.* Healthcare Quality Quest, Romsey.

Donabedian A (1980) *Definition of Quality and Approaches to its Assessment.* Health Administration Press, Ann Arbor, Michigan.

Etzioni A (1969) *The Semi-Professions and their Organisations.* Free Press, London.

Irvine D (1998) *General Medical Council News.* GMC, London.

Leape LL, Brennan TA, Laird N *et al.* (1991) The nature of adverse events in hospitalised patients. Results of Harvard Medical Practice Study II. *New England Journal of Medicine.* **324**: 377–84.

MDU (1999) The future of medical liability in Europe. *Journal of MDU.* **15**.

Mills DH (ed) (1977) *Report on the Medical Insurance Feasibility Study.* California Medical Association, San Francisco, CA.

Murrell G, Huang C and Ellis H (1999) *Research in Medicine* (2e). Cambridge University Press, Cambridge.

Nolan, Lord (1995) *Standards in Public Life: first report of the Committee on Standards in Public Life.* HMSO, London.

NHSE (1999) *Faster Access to Modern Treatment: how NICE appraisal will work.* NHS Executive, Leeds.

NHSE (1999) *Clinical Governance: quality in the new NHS* (HSC 1999/0065). The Stationery Office, London.

Sackett DL, Rosenberg WMC, Gray JAM and Haynes RB (1996) Evidence-based medicine: what it is and what it isn't. *BMJ.* **312**: 71–2.

Scally G and Donaldson LJ (1998) Clinical governance and the drive for quality improvement in the new NHS in England. *BMJ.* **317**: 61–5.

Shaw CD and Costain DW (1989) Guidelines for medical audit: seven principles. *BMJ.* **299**: 498–9.

Stevens A, Colin-Jones D and Gabbay J (1995) Quick and clean: authoritative health technology assessment for local health care contracting. *Health Trends.* **27**: 37–42.

Thompson R (1996) Quality in health care. In: A White (ed) *Textbook of Management for Doctors.* Churchill Livingstone, Edinburgh.

Taylor DG (1998) *Improving Health Care.* King's Fund Policy Paper 2. King's Fund, London.

Wilson R, Runciman WB, Gibberd RW *et al.* (1995) The Quality in Australian Health Care Study. *Medical Journal of Australia.* **163**: 458–71.

7

Understanding the NHS

The aim of this chapter is to provide an outline of recent reforms and an understanding of the structure of the NHS, both nationally and locally. It also reviews healthcare reforms in a worldwide context and current thinking about hospitals of the future.

A statistical picture of the NHS

- Every day, nearly 700 000 people visit their general practitioner and about 100 000 visit their dentist.
- Every day, over 1700 babies are delivered.
- A one-week stay in hospital costs £1100 and a night in intensive care costs £500.
- Over 559 million prescriptions are dispensed each year, costing £5000 million. This represents 12% of all NHS expenditure.
- The NHS UK budget is just over £46 billion (when it started in 1948 it was £400 million). This represents over £1000 every second.
- 77% of funding comes from general taxation, 12% from the NHS share of national insurance contributions and 2% from patient charges.
- Just under half of NHS spending goes on acute services. This amounts to about £800 per person per annum.
- The NHS spends £14 billion in Scotland and £7 billion in Wales.
- Over 40% of total hospital and community health services expenditure is for people over 64 years of age, though they represent just 16% of the population.
- About 5.6% of the gross domestic product is spent on healthcare, placing the UK 17th out of 22 OECD countries.
- The NHS employs nearly one million people (7.5% of all UK employment) and is Europe's largest civilian employer.
- Staff costs account for two-thirds of all expenditure.

The new NHS structure

The NHS provides care via various routes.

- Primary care through family doctors, opticians, dentists and other healthcare professionals.
- Secondary care through hospitals and ambulance services.
- Tertiary care through specialist hospitals treating particular types of illness such as cancer.
- Community care through partnership with local social services departments.

The NHS went through considerable change when the Labour entered government in 1997. These changes were set out in the White Paper, *The New NHS*, published in December of that year and accompanied by papers for Scotland, Wales and Northern Ireland. The main commitment was to replace the internal market with a system based on co-operation and partnership. In England this meant essentially two key things: retaining separation between health authorities and trusts and replacing GP fundholding with primary care groups and trusts.

The New NHS is based on six principles:

- a national service
- delivery against national standards, and local responsibility
- characterised by partnership, not competition
- efficiency through a rigorous approach to performance and cutting bureaucracy
- moving the focus on to excellence and quality
- rebuilding public confidence in the NHS.

Although co-operation and partnership were stressed, competition did not disappear entirely, as PCG/Ts are still able to choose which NHS trust provides care for their patients. Data published about performance seeks to ensure that competition is by comparative results.

This chapter describes some of the major players in the NHS hierarchy and how they relate to each other. You need to be aware, however, that details change. The one continuing feature has been change in the balance between central and local control.

The Department of Health

Overall responsibility for the NHS in England lies with the Secretary of State for Health. Supported by the Department of Health in London, one of the biggest Whitehall Departments, the Secretary of State sets the strategic direction for the NHS and answers to Parliament. The Secretary of State (often referred to as the

Health Secretary) is supported by two ministers of state and two parliamentary under-secretaries of state who have defined responsibilities for aspects of the Department's work.

The Department is organised into three areas, the most important of which is the NHS Executive. The other two are the public health and social care groups. There are four agencies responsible for particular functions: the Medical Devices Agency, the Medicine Control Agency, the NHS Pensions Agency, and the NHS Estates Agency.

There is a permanent secretary (a senior civil servant) in the Department who advises the Secretary of State. The Chief Executive of the NHS Executive is directly accountable to the Secretary of State for managing the NHS. The Chief Medical Officer is the government's chief medical advisor and is responsible to the Secretary of State for medical matters. There are also other senior civil servants including the Chief Nursing Officer, Chief Dental Officer, Chief Pharmaceutical Officer and Chief Social Services Inspector.

Responsibility for NHS policy and operation lies with the NHS Executive, a part of the Department of Health with its headquarters in Leeds, and eight regional offices each with a regional director. The Executive implements health policies laid down by the Secretary of State and manages the funding and the way the service operates.

Parliament is responsible for voting resources to the NHS and holds the Secretary of State accountable for resources used. Health authorities, trusts, and PCG/Ts may be required to provide information and data to the Department to enable issues raised in Parliament to be answered. Parliamentary select committees reinforce this scrutiny.

NHS Policy Board

This Board is responsible for strategy and is chaired by the Secretary of State for Health. It includes non-executive members drawn from inside and outside the NHS.

NHS Executive (NHSE)

Originally the NHS Management Executive (NHSME), the NHSE sets the policy framework for the NHS, and is the biggest business area within the Department of Health. Its headquarters are situated in Leeds and there are eight regional offices. It is made up of a chief executive, regional directors and directors of headquarter functions such as human resources, planning and finance.

NHSE Regional Offices

These replace the old regional health authorities and are smaller organisations, each headed by a regional director. Regional offices monitor financial performance in NHS trusts and review annual reports and accounts. They also examine trusts' annual business plans, which set out capital investment and service development proposals.

Health authorities

Each health authority covers a population of about 500 000. These authorities comprise a non-executive chairman appointed by the Health Secretary and a board of executive and non-executive directors. There are usually five non-executive directors, and the executive team includes a chief executive, finance director and director of public health. Their role is to provide strategic leadership at local level and are required to carry out assessment of local health needs and to develop plans to meet these needs through a health improvement programme (HImP) (*see* Chapter 6).

Special health authorities

There are over a dozen special health authorities. Each has a unique function and some have remits which extend beyond England. They include the National Blood Authority, the NHS Litigation Authority, the NHS Information Authority, the Health Education Authority and the National Institute for Clinical Excellence.

Specialist regional and supraregional services

New arrangements have been introduced for planning and commissioning services that are only required at regional or national level because of their complexity, cost or level of incidence. It includes in-service agreements, which are planned through advisory groups and provided by nominated specialist providers.

Public Accounts Committee

This Committee scrutinises the way in which money voted by parliament is spent. It is supported by the comptroller, auditor general and the National Audit Office.

The chief executive of the NHS may be called before the Committee to answer questions.

Health Select Committee

This Committee complements the work of the Public Accounts Committee and shadows the work of the Department, carrying out inquiries into major health policy issues.

Select Committee on the Parliamentary Commissioner for Administration

This Committee follows up reports of the health service commissioner or ombudsman who is responsible for investigating areas of maladministration in the NHS, failure to provide a service and other complaints from the public.

The Audit Commission

An independent body set up by Parliament which takes an interest in auditing the NHS with particular reference to value for money.

National Institute for Clinical Excellence (NICE)

See Chapter 6.

Commission for Health Improvement (CHI)

See Chapter 6.

General Medical Council (GMC)

The GMC is a statutory body that is primarily concerned with medical registration and ensuring practising doctors meet certain specified standards. The GMC assesses evidence of continuing education, professional development and standards of performance through the revalidation process.

Community health councils (CHC)

CHCs were statutory bodies established in 1974 as a consumer voice in the NHS. Voluntary organisations, local authorities and the local community nominated members. A typical budget would be around £50 000. Although they enjoyed no powers, they did have rights of access to information, to consultation, etc. They were intended to advise health authorities on the views and concerns of patients and the public.

CHCs are to be abolished from March 2002 and replaced by local advisory forums, supported by patients' forums, local authority scrutiny committees and patient advocacy and liaison roles established by trusts.

NHS Litigation Authority (NHSLA)

In the past, NHS trusts took out commercial insurance to cover for a wide range of non-clinical risks. The increasing costs of successful clinical negligence claims led to the establishment of the Clinical Negligence Scheme for Trusts (CNST) which is now administered by the NHSLA. More than 80% of NHS trusts insure their clinical risk this way.

The NHS in England

Devolution has had significant implications for the structure and provision of health services across the UK as Wales and Scotland have assumed responsibility for a wide range of services. Westminster has retained UK-wide power only over the following:

- abortion
- human fertilisation
- human genetics
- xenotransplantation
- regulation of medicines.

The NHS in Scotland has a budget of £14 billion and Wales £7 billion. Scotland also has tax varying powers although Wales has not. Scotland spends 30% more per capita and Wales 15% more, than England.

The NHS in Scotland

There have always been differences between the English and Scottish health services and the variations in approach are reflected in the White Paper for Scotland, *Designed to Care*. The main differences relate to primary care. Primary care trusts (PCTs) came into force in Scotland in April 1999 and are responsible for the full range of services including mental health services. Their organisation reflects the local healthcare co-operatives and voluntary organisations formed by general practitioners.

Scottish PCTs do not generally commission secondary care, partly due to the fact that there was less interest in fundholding in Scotland. They have, however, developed the joint investment fund (JIF).

From July 1999, the Scottish Executive, headed by its First Minister, was responsible and accountable to the Scottish Parliament for the NHS in Scotland. Scottish ministers are accountable to that Parliament for the development and delivery of services. There is a Management Executive with 15 health boards responsible for planning and commissioning hospital and community services as well as managing primary care services. There are 35 trusts, each accountable to the Scottish Minister via the Management Executive.

The NHS in Wales

During 1999, all the health responsibilities of the Welsh Office passed to the National Assembly for Wales. The Assembly is led by the First Secretary, with the Department for Health being the responsibility of the under-secretary. The NHS in Wales is headed by a director, who is supported by a Chief Medical Officer for Wales.

There are 19 trusts in Wales. For primary care, local health groups (LHG) were set up broadly coterminous with the 22 unitary authorities. LHGs are committees of health authorities and advise them.

The NHS in Northern Ireland

There were 19 health and social services trusts and five GP commissioning group pilot schemes as of April 1999. Due to changing circumstances surrounding the political situation, the relationship between the Northern Ireland Assembly and healthcare provision remains unclear.

Primary care

Nine out of ten people are seen in the community, which is why the community doctor or GP is said to be the cornerstone of the NHS. Everyone has the right to be registered with a GP. In addition to providing primary care, GPs also act as 'gatekeepers' to the rest of the service, referring patients where appropriate to hospital or specialist treatment. There are 35 500 GPs, mostly working in groups, and the typical GP has a list of 1900 patients. There are also about 15 000 dentists.

Primary healthcare teams generally deal with every patient and must cope with many simultaneous demands and pressures. Expectations or treatment goals for groups of people with chronic disease need to be clear and success or failure of chronic disease treatment often depends on the patient's contribution. They need to be motivated, have sufficient understanding of their condition and their individual life circumstances should be taken into account in agreed management plans. There needs to be clear guidance on referral. Primary carers do not want their patients trapped in secondary or even tertiary care.

The introduction of performance-related contracts during the early 1990s encouraged many GPs to run health promotion clinics and carry out minor surgery, as well as improve immunisation rates. In addition to GPs, other healthcare professionals provide a range of primary care services. These include dentists, physiotherapists, opticians, pharmacists, health visitors, midwives, community nurses, occupational therapists and speech therapists.

In April 1999, all GPs and community nurses became members of primary care groups. There are 480 such groups covering populations ranging from 46 000 to 257 000 patients. Each PCG is overseen by a board comprised of four to seven GPs, up to two community or practice nurses, a social services nominee, a lay member, a health authority non-executive and the chief executive. The board is accountable through the chief executive to the health authority.

PCGs are committees of health authorities and have three main roles:

- to improve the health of the community
- to develop primary and community services
- to commission secondary care services.

Health authorities (HAs) have to support the development of PCG/Ts, enabling them to take increasing responsibility so that they can become free-standing bodies or primary care trusts.

PCGs may choose to operate at one of the following levels:

- Level 1: as an advisory sub-committee of the HA
- Level 2: as a budget holding sub-committee of the HA
- Level 3: a PCT taking responsibility for commissioning hospital and community health services

• Level 4: a PCT which in addition can provide community health services.

Mergers and movement towards trust status are seen as inevitable developments by most PCGs.

Secondary care

• Most secondary care is provided by hospitals operating as trusts.
• Around 375 trusts manage more than 98% of all NHS hospitals and community health services.
• There are around 280 major district general hospitals in England.
• Between 1984 and 1996, the number of beds for all specialties fell from about 335 000 to 212 000, while the number of in-patient cases treated rose by more than a third.
• In excess of 12 million patients are treated in A&E services each year.
• The average length of hospital stay is eight days (1995); this compares to 45 days in 1951.
• The average overnight bed occupancy is 81.2% (1996/7).

Secondary care organisations seek to be responsive, provide a comprehensive service and communicate well to meet the needs of patients and their GPs. At tertiary level, services focus on providing specialised service for which they alone may have the skills.

NHS trusts

Trusts are independent organisations within the NHS. They may be a single hospital, a group of hospitals, community services provided in health centres and clinics, an ambulance service, or a primary care trust. There are some 375 NHS trusts in England. Trusts were first established in 1991 under the NHS reforms of the previous year. They are self-governing service providers within the NHS and each has its own trust board comprised of executive and non-executive directors. The chair is appointed by the Secretary of State and they in turn appoint five non-executive directors, bringing expertise and ideas from a range of backgrounds and professions, and providing a link with local communities. The trust board is then responsible for appointing the management board which consists of five executive directors – this must include a chief executive, a medical director, a senior nurse and a finance director. The major district general hospitals provide services from A&E to the care of elderly people.

NHS trusts have full responsibility for operational management. The income they receive comes from service agreements negotiated with health authorities and PCG/Ts rather than annual contracts. In addition to a statutory duty of quality of care they are accountable to the NHS Executive for their statutory duty to break even financially. They also have to work within a framework of HImPs and contribute to developing these programmes. They are also required to work in partnership with health authorities.

The four most typical models are:

- acute hospital trusts, mostly district general hospitals, but some single specialty units also exist
- integrated service trusts, providing acute and community services and, in some cases, also mental health services
- mental health trusts, sometimes with services for people with learning disabilities
- primary care trusts.

Trusts are directly accountable to the Secretary of State via the regional offices of the NHS Executive, which monitor performance. The trust board makes decisions about policy and strategic direction. The statutory basis for the board is contained in the National Health Service Trusts (Membership and Procedure) Regulations 1990 (Statutory Instrument 1990, No. 2024).

Trusts' statutory powers include:

- setting up their own management structure subject to national requirements regarding the involvement of senior professional staff
- employing staff on terms and conditions set by the trust
- buying and selling property
- borrowing money, within annually agreed limits – primarily for capital developments
- entering into NHS and other contracts
- generating income, subject to this not interfering with other obligations.

NHS trusts do not receive direct financial allocations but operate on an income and expenditure basis. Sources of income derive from agreements to provide services for health authorities and primary care organisations; undergraduate medical and dental education; postgraduate medical education; education and training for other healthcare professionals; carrying out medical research; and from other services such as car parking and hospital shops.

Non-executive directors

There are currently about 3000 people serving as non-executive directors of healthcare trusts. They are 'the voice of the local community' and should normally live in the area served by the trust. They normally devote about three days a month to trust responsibilities either during the working day or in the evening. Their primary task is to safeguard the public interest. They are accountable to the health authority (or health board in Scotland) and are supposed to work within the spirit of Lord Nolan's (1995) seven principles of public life: selflessness, integrity, objectivity, accountability, openness, honesty and leadership.

As well as visiting hospitals, health centres, general practices and other sites in their locality, they are given training opportunities to increase their skills and understanding of their work. They are appointed for an initial period of up to four years. Appointments are renewable, although change is encouraged.

The person specification drawn up for selection includes the following essential qualities. The person should:

- live in the area served by the trust
- have a strong personal commitment to the NHS
- demonstrate a commitment to the needs of the local community
- be a good communicator with plenty of common sense
- be committed to the public service values of accountability, probity, openness and equality of opportunity
- demonstrate ability to contribute to the work of the board
- be available for about three days per month
- demonstrate an interest in healthcare issues.

It is also regarded as desirable that they:

- have experience as a carer or user of the NHS
- have experience of serving in the voluntary sector
- have served the local community in local government or some other capacity
- understand or have experience of management in the public, private or voluntary sectors
- offer specialist skills or knowledge relevant to the work of the trust.

Applications are encouraged from all sections of the community, particularly women, people from ethnic minorities and people with disabilities. Political activity should not be a consideration in selection and information on political activity is requested on application forms for monitoring purposes only.

Non-executive directors work with four or five other non-executives and the senior trust managers, including the medical director, as equal members of the trust board. They are expected to use their personal skills and experience of the community and the NHS to guide the trust in the following areas:

- developing long-term plans for healthcare in the local community
- best use of its financial resources to help patients
- appointment of chief executive and other senior managers
- various committees such as the:

- Remuneration Committee to ensure fair pay for trust executives
- Audit Committee to ensure proper financial procedures
- committees to review professional conduct and staff discipline matters
- ensuring the trust meets its commitment to the Patient's Charter and other targets
- contributing to the relationship between the trust and the local community and media by representing the board at official occasions
- overseeing the trust's response to complaints from the public
- being involved in hearing appeals by patients detained under the Mental Health Act.

Non-executive directors are paid £5000 per annum and they may claim travel and subsistence costs while on trust business. Conflicts of interest with commercial, public or voluntary bodies have to be declared and these are published in an annual report with details of all board members' remuneration from NHS sources.

Chairs of NHS trusts

A trust chair must have the same qualities as a non-executive director and, in addition, be able to demonstrate leadership and motivation skills, the ability to think strategically and the ability to understand complex issues. Management experience at a senior level in the public, private or voluntary sectors is seen as a desirable attribute.

The chair is accountable to the Secretary of State for giving leadership to the NHS trust board and to ensure that, through the chief executive, the trust achieves the following:

- provides efficient and effective healthcare and health education services to the community
- collaborates with the regional chairman and the regional office of the NHS Executive to implement national and local policies trust
- works with GPs, health authorities and local authority social services departments to plan and deliver integrated services
- maintains financial viability, using resources effectively, and controls and reports its finances within guidelines issued by the NHS Executive
- meets legal and contractual obligations by carrying out statutory responsibilities with due regard to relevant EC directives, requirements of statutory bodies, hazard or safety notices, advice relating to patient, public or staff safety and personal privacy and patient confidentiality
- undertakes, commissions or makes facilities available for research and plays a part in medical education as appropriate, in conjunction with medical schools and research funding bodies
- co-operates and develops links with the community

• promotes actively the values and achievements of the NHS.

The chair generally devotes around three days a week to trust duties, for which he or she is paid between £15125–£19285 per annum, depending on the size of the trust.

Action

- Consider the background and possible value and input of non-executive directors for your trust.
- Who are the non-executive directors in your trust?
- List any meetings they chair or contribute to.
- What is their background?
- What do you think they might bring to the job?
- What is the chair's leadership style?
- How do they relate to the professionals in the trust?

Clinical directorates

In parallel with the constant flux in the balance of control between central government and local arrangements, there has been a steady move towards involvement of hospital doctors in organisational management. This has now been extended to primary care. Parliament continues to seek to hold the medical profession more accountable for standards and for contribution to overall performance through the new arrangements to improve quality.

The move to devolve policy has been accompanied by devolution of resources and processes to staff delivering the care, while maintaining corporate control and accountability. Each separate sub-unit has contractual obligations and, where possible, a single person accountable for performance.

If led by a clinician these units are generally known as 'clinical directorates', or 'business units' where they are led by managers, although terms and structures vary between hospitals. The Griffiths' report stated, 'The nearer the management process gets to the patient, the more important it becomes for the doctors to be looked upon as the natural managers'.

A trust's management team is responsible for the operational management and the development of policy within the trust. The management team is made up of the executive directors and the clinical directors of the trust. Clinical directors are usually consultant medical staff, although occasionally they may be a professional other than a doctor. They are accountable to the chief executive for the management of patient care and treatment involving clinical staff in the development and management of services.

The key elements of the clinical director's role fall under the day-to-day general management headings, and include:

- responsibility for the directorate budget, manpower and staffing
- clinical services including clinical audit and management
- budget management and control
- business and strategic planning
- services planning, service development, strategic development, staff development, business development, and clinical development of the trust.

There are usually several clinical directorates within each trust, working alongside others to provide the services required. This number varies considerably according to the size of the trust but, generally, there are around eight clinical directorates per trust, although in a few instances have reached as many as 30.

Issues for clinical directorates include the development of future patterns of service, medical staffing issues, coping with pressures (particularly in emergency admissions), reorganisations, transfers, mergers, rationalisation and waiting lists.

Action

Draw an organisational chart setting out the location of titles such as clinical director, medical director, chief executive, finance director, human resource director and others within your trust.

- To whom is the clinical director accountable? The medical director or chief executive?
- What is the clinical director responsible for?
- Is the business manager accountable to the clinical director or chief executive?
- Ask about the difference between operational and strategic management.
- Who decides strategy in your hospital?
- What are the links between the trust strategy and patient care?

It might be helpful to look through the section on key reports and publications in Chapter 9, which gives a brief outline of some of the key legislation and reports in this area.

Community care

The NHS spends about £4 billion annually on medicines and around 10 000 pharmacies dispense over 400 million prescriptions annually. Over 80% of these are dispensed free of charge.

The NHS also plays an important role in providing community care services to meet the needs of the elderly, those with disabilities, the mentally ill and other frail or vulnerable members of society. Social service departments of local councils take the lead role for community care and the NHS is responsible for working with them to ensure the effective planning and delivery of community care services. This involves contributing to the assessment of people's needs for community care, liaising over hospital discharge for those requiring continuing support, as well as delivering services.

Since the introduction of community care reforms in 1993, the lead responsibility for community care has rested with social service departments. Working closely with the NHS, housing authorities and other agencies, they are responsible for planning, co-ordinating and assessing individual need for community care services. The aim of the community care reforms was to ensure that services are more effectively tailored to meet the needs and preferences of individuals. While not appropriate in every case, the emphasis is on supporting people in their own homes or in homely community settings where feasible and sensible.

The NHS makes an important contribution to meeting needs for community care. For instance, district nurses provide 2.3 million episodes of care annually, and over one million chiropody sessions are carried out in the home. Recent guidance has confirmed and clarified the NHS's responsibilities for meeting continuing healthcare needs and all health authorities have been required to publish local policies and eligibility criteria for continuing healthcare, giving details of local services.

Shared care

Shared care is not about a relationship between one doctor and one patient. Rather, it is about multiple relationships to treat a disease or condition, involving contributions from the patient and a range of healthcare providers. The objective of healthcare is to achieve a satisfactory clinical outcome within available resources. Increasingly, healthcare professionals work as teams. Surgical and medical teams have different needs, the latter in particular may not only be multi-disciplinary but also distributed between primary and secondary healthcare. Conditions which are relatively common and susceptible to timely appropriate interventions are often managed by fragmented and unco-ordinated services. Such conditions tend to require primary care services, specialised secondary care services and, sometimes, highly specialised secondary care – and a few require highly specialised tertiary care.

Integrated care

PCG/Ts and health authorities have a responsibility for ensuring that patients within the area have a service that meets their needs. A major challenge is commissioning for a service that is met by a variety of providers – in primary care, in the community, in local trusts and some in more distant regional centres. Developments in the provision of diabetic services provide a useful example of emerging approaches which include:

- diabetes centre representatives (medical, nursing and relevant professions allied to medicine)
- primary care representatives (medical and nursing)
- community representatives (medical, nursing and relevant professions allied to medicine)
- director of public health or manager
- patient representatives
- specialist representatives as required.

Integrated care is a logical way to approach the management of chronic diseases. Models vary according to local needs and cultures.

Healthcare reforms

Before leaving government and the NHS reforms, it might be helpful to consider healthcare in a global context. In the quest for improved efficiency, policy makers worldwide have introduced a range of healthcare reforms which seek to contain costs, increase efficiency and raise standards. There are no quick-fix solutions to the challenges faced by healthcare systems in developed countries.

The experiences of five different countries have been reviewed, chosen for their different systems of finance and delivery. In Holland and Germany, social insurance is the predominant method of funding with a mixed economy of public and private providers. The UK and Sweden pay for healthcare mainly out of taxation, with a large measure of public ownership of hospitals and public employment of staff. The US relies mainly on private funding and provision, using competition to increase efficiency and promote choice for patients.

Four approaches to reform can be identified.

1 **Big Bang**   Reform introduced in a short period of time and driven through by a government committed to its implementation. This has occurred in the UK, Israel and New Zealand.
2 **Incremental reform**   This tends to be a lengthy process with key proposals not being implemented after a period of 10 years. This has occurred in Holland and Germany.
3 **Bottom-up reform**   A number of national policy initiatives set by local councils, as in Sweden.
4 **Reform without reform**   Rapid changes occurring continuously despite the defeat of central plans, as in US and, partly, Sweden.

The way in which reforms are implemented is also interesting. It may be as a broad outline with the detail added at a later stage, as with the recent NHS reforms. Generally in other countries too the implementation stage is important. Key aspects of the original proposal may be adapted at a decentralised level and the content and direction of the reforms shaped locally. Policies can also create politics. For example, policies developed in one period can give rise to a set of relationships between organisations and interested parties in the healthcare system, which in turn shapes the development of future policies.

The NHS of the future

During the pilot stages of the first edition of this book we were frequently asked to include a section on the future of the NHS. We claim no crystal ball and have no more insight than any other person working in healthcare. The glib answer is to state that you (the intended readers) are the future, but to fulfil our promise to take notice of all comments at the pilot stages we have set out some of the developments that are on the horizon and could well develop in the future.

If you feel that change is a new issue you need look no further than *The Principles and Practice of Medicine* by William Osler (1895) who wrote over 100 years ago, 'Everywhere the old order changes and happy those who change with it.'

There exist technological forces for change, such as minimally invasive therapies, diagnostic scanning techniques, microchip technology, advances in biotechnical diagnostic testing, more finely targeted drugs, together with new drug delivery systems and, perhaps, routine genetic therapy. Social changes must be taken into account in both the domestic and working environment. Cultural shift caused by societal, individual, political or professional change has tended to decentralise power and influence, and increased user involvement in policy making leads to different expectations of healthcare. Resource developments in primary care create further pressure for change in the structure of provision. Increasing patient expectations and patient autonomy, together with the information revolution that allows individuals greater access to global information, will be drivers for change in the responsiveness of professionals. There is also rising demand due to ageing as well as medical advances.

One recent medical advance is 'telemedicine' where a patient consults the doctor from home via a video link, which incorporates special sensors to relay vital signs. One can also imagine robotic surgeons – controlled by experts on the other side of the world – operating on patients within the next decade. The telephone can be used to monitor the heart, as patients are now able to send a 30-second recording for analysis by a doctor. Follow-up telephone consultations at pre-agreed times to discuss progress mean that patients don't have to journey to the out-patients department, and the results of one such example – in rheumatology – have already been published. Certain specialties such as rheumatology, dermatology and neurology are more suited to this approach, and some centres are already carrying out post-operative follow-ups, particularly for day surgery patients.

NHS Direct, the telephone help-line, is now firmly established. Staffed by nurses, NHS Direct provides medical advice and reassurance to reduce the number of unnecessary ambulance call-outs, hospital attendance and out-of-hours GP call-outs.

Nursing units with nurses running their own hospitals are another possible future development. Hospices and specialised units for Aids are already taking medical innovation into new territory. Hospital-at-home schemes already cater for renal dialysis, IV therapy and nutrition, respiratory therapy, intensive nursing, rehabilitation therapy and obstetrics.

Not only will the buildings change but the organisation, staff and management will too. Evidence-based management built on good research evidence and appropriate use of limited resources will require managers to have an understanding of key clinical issues. This will all be part of the development of more methodical approaches to risk management and quality, as enshrined in clinical governance. The Commission for Health Improvement has established a rolling programme of reviews of NHS trust performance, ensuring that clinical standards are maintained. NICE publishes guidelines on the most clinically-effective and cost-effective treatments and drugs. Clinical pathways are developed for optimal sequencing and timing of interventions by clinicians, nurses and allied healthcare workers – a firm move away from 'cook book' medicine. Hospitals are now required to publish detailed league tables and data, and mortality and morbidity leagues are now beginning to appear.

We may also see a continuing move away from professional self-regulation towards more direct accountability. Indeed, since the previous edition there have been dramatic changes in the GMC's role and the introduction of revalidation for continued registration of all doctors.

The careers of consultants will change as the position will no longer represent the pinnacle for hospital doctors. Having reached consultant-level they will have various branches to follow: towards clinical director in service work, teaching, research or management; medical director and even chief executive. Doctors' roles in management will continue to develop as interested parties demand that doctors fulfil their roles with skill.

As Plato said, quoting Protagoras in the fifth century, 'Of all things the measure is man: of things that are, that they are, and of things that are not, that they are not.' Staffing will remain the key, for even with the most sophisticated and technical advances there will always be the need for human contact. There will be staffing changes as well as changes in staff and there are already shortages of both nurses and doctors. Adequate staffing levels may, however, be interpreted and reacted to differently by governments, patients and healthcare professionals.

Related reading

Beware when reading anything further about the NHS's structure. It changes frequently and anything more than a year old is very likely to be out of date.

Beverley N (1997) NHS trusts and provision of health services. In: *NAHAT NHS Handbook 1997/98.* Section 2.6, Overview of Finances and Accountability.

Croner (2000) *Croner's Health Service Manager.* Croner Publications, Kingston-upon-Thames. Also available on disk. An excellent data source of material in this section.

Ham C (1999) *The Organisation of the NHS.* In: *Wellard's NHS Handbook 1999/2000.* Section 1.2. Sets one's own organisation within the context of the NHS. It's also a useful overview of the recent years of NHS reforms.

NHSE (1995) *Priorities and Planning Guidance for the NHS: 1999/2000.* NHS Executive, Leeds. Part 1 covers strategic purpose and results, the purpose of the NHS, policies of the NHS, baseline requirements and objectives, medium-term priorities and the local planning context. Part 2 covers objective setting for 1999/2000 and milestones for medium-term priorities.

Nolan, Lord (1995) *Standards in Public Life: first report of the committee on standards in public life.* HMSO, London.

Wall A (1999) NHS boards and their functions. In: *Wellard's NHS Handbook 1999/2000.* Useful on the role of non-executive directors. There is also something on this in Croner's *Health Service Manager.*

8

Funding and the NHS

The aim of this chapter is to inform you about national and local NHS funding structures.

The finances of the NHS

National level financing

Government sets spending levels after balancing the needs expressed by the Department of Health and NHSE and the requirements of HM Treasury, set within governmental economic and political priorities.

The main source of funds is general taxation, which accounts for 77% of income. 12% comes from the NHS part of National Insurance Contributions and 2% from patient charges. The remainder comes from capital refunds to trusts (8%) and miscellaneous sources (1%).

Distribution of NHS funds

Funding supports the Department of Health, hospital, community and family health services, and centrally purchased services such as the National Blood Authority.

The basis for distributing the total NHS funds varies between England, Wales, Scotland and Northern Ireland, and at national and regional level part of the NHS budget is top-sliced to fund special initiatives and regional office expenses. The remainder is distributed direct to health authorities.

Allocations to health authorities

These comprise three main elements:

- baseline allocation relating to previous year
- allocation for inflation
- real increase varying in amount according to an authority's distance from target in relation to 'fair shares target'.

Health authorities may not overdraw their allocation but are allowed to carry forward planned under-spending without limit, although they are not encouraged to do so.

Every year, following the Chancellor's Budget statement, each health authority is allocated a share of the available resources according to a national formula. A unified budget incorporates hospital, community and general medical services. GP prescribing is cash-limited.

Capital in the NHS

Formerly a government funded capital grant, but now a mix of two elements: governmental funding (reflected in costs and prices) and the private finance initiative (PFI) (with revenue costs).

The Private Finance Initiative (PFI)

This was intended to give the NHS (and other public sector organisations) access to private sector skills and expertise, as well as being a source of finance for capital investment. Under PFI, private sector finance has been used to improve the NHS in a range of areas, in both clinical and support services such as clinical waste incineration.

Each case for major capital spending (of over £10m) is subject to a strategic review or development strategy and an outline business case. If outline approval is granted then a full business case is prepared for approval by the regional office, NHSE and, for schemes over £50m, HM Treasury ministers.

The National Audit Office (NAO)

Headed by the Comptroller and Auditor General, the NAO is the external auditor of central government spending in the UK. Established under the *National Audit Act*

1983, the NAO's role is to ensure accountability to Parliament and the taxpayer for all moneys voted by Parliament. The Comptroller and Auditor General also have statutory powers to certify a wide range of public sector accounts, and statutory powers to report to Parliament on the economic efficiency and effectiveness with which departments and other bodies have used their resources.

The NAO publishes about 50 value for money reports each year, including five covering the work of the Department of Health and the NHSE.

The Accounts Commission for Scotland

This is a statutory independent body that assists the NHS (and local government) in Scotland to achieve high standards of financial stewardship and value for money. It secures external audit of all Scottish health service bodies and reports concerns identified through audit which are followed up by statutory power where appropriate. Copies of reports can be downloaded from their website.

Finances at local level

Trusts obtain most of their income through service agreements or commissions with health authorities and PCG/Ts. These agreements set out the treatment or services the trust agrees to provide in return for funding. Agreements can include quality clauses and requirements to meet targets for equal opportunities, respond to complaints and provide information to the public. Trusts have the power to make investment decisions for themselves and, with their financial freedom, can develop services for patients. The trust has only a single financial obligation – to break even. Details of the ways in which trusts obtain income are set out fully in Chapter 7.

Financial control within NHS trusts

Members of trust boards have to ensure that the trust:

- publishes a strategic direction document every third year covering the next five-year period
- publishes a summary business plan by 31 March each year
- ensures that the annual income and expenditure budget is realistic
- makes adequate provision for inflation
- receives a monthly report showing financial position with forecast of year end position
- organises its management in an effective manner within limits set by the NHSE.

Trusts must comply with certain requirements in pricing their services:

- prices must equal costs for NHS agreements
- costs must include depreciation and a 6% return on the value of assets employed
- there must be no cross subsidising between services
- marginal costs can only be charged where unplanned spare capacity exists
- for private contracts charges should be what the market will bear.

Most hospital service agreements, and consequently most income, are for clinical services – those clinical services therefore have to recover in their prices a fair proportion of the full cost to the hospital, rather than simply their direct costs.

Top-down cost allocation is a well-established process whereby overhead or central costs, such as for estates services, general management, finance and personnel, are apportioned over the clinical support and patient care departments, usually on the basis of some surrogate data such as floor area or head count. The clinical support departments, for example anaesthetics, HDU, pathology and radiology, are then apportioned to each directorate on the basis of use and added to the costs of wards and theatres to establish the directorate's total costs. The result of this process is to absorb the whole cost of the hospital into the clinical directorates. The impact is that while the direct costs of a directorate may be, say, £1 million, its fully absorbed costs may be double that or more. Since accurate usage data are seldom available, the apportionment of costs to directorates is sometimes a matter of considerable debate.

The relative prices of treatments within a directorate are established through bottom-up costing. This should involve clinical staff in broadly defining care profiles for each treatment. The profiles incorporating length of stay, nursing dependency, theatres and other key resources should concentrate on the major elements of cost rather than on what may be clinically significant but of low cost. Once all treatments have an agreed profile for costing, these are used as weights applied to the planned numbers of patients to absorb the full cost to the directorate. It should also be noted that hospitals also usually take account of the prices charged for similar procedures in other hospitals within the region.

Service agreements

The previous internal market has been replaced with service agreements setting out the responsibility of both parties on cost, volume, quality, efficiency and effectiveness of service, often with three to five year agreements being sought.

Out of area treatments (OAT)

As the internal market was abolished it became necessary to replace extra-contractual referrals with a new system that avoided cumbersome billing.

National Schedule of Referenced Costs (NSRC)

Part of the government's approach to tackling poor standards in relation to costs is to require trusts to publish their costs on a consistent basis, covering all surgical in-patient and day cases together with some medical specialties.

The costs are aggregated at national level and published as an index. The aim is to allow meaningful discussion between health authorities, PCG/Ts and NHS trusts. These reference costs are also part of a national framework for assessing performance.

Primary care groups and trusts (PCG/T)

All GPs must belong to one of the 481 PCGs in England (effectively functioning as sub-groups of the health authority), which may operate in one of four ways:

- Level One (advisory): at minimum, advising the health authority on commissioning care
- Level Two (managing delegated budget): managing the budget for all healthcare in their area in tandem with the health authority
- Level Three (PCTs accountable for commissioning): as free-standing commissioning bodies accountable to the health authority
- Level Four (PCTs): as above, but with added responsibility for community services.

Accountability runs between the chair of the PCG (usually a GP) and the chief executive of the health authority. The chair also manages the chief executive of the PCG and is accountable for the budget.

In Wales, local health groups have been established which are coterminous with unitary authorities and have broader representation with elected representatives. In Scotland integrated PCTs have been established, supported by local GP co-operatives. The degree of engagement of GPs is different in the three countries, with England having more freedom and direct engagement. As the national assemblies develop, these differences are likely to increase.

Health commissioning

When the NHS internal market and GP fundholding were abolished, health authorities and PCG/Ts became responsible for commissioning services. The roles of health authorities (and health boards in Scotland) are, therefore, evolving and each of the four countries have adopted their own approach. The emphasis is on primary care and increasing its involvement in and responsibility for commissioning, with health authorities expected to play a strategic and supporting role. NHS trusts are anxious about the potential erosion of their autonomy. It is thought that the influence of health authorities may decrease over time as PCG/Ts assume responsibility for commissioning.

The role of health authorities has to some extent diminished with the development of locality-based commissioning. They have taken on a more strategic role in local service configuration in order to address the wider public health agenda and health inequalities. Health authorities take a specific lead in initiating strategic change, allocating health resources, quality control and acting as a counterbalance to parochial agendas.

The stated purpose of health authorities is to make the best use of available resources to improve health and prevent illness by influencing other organisations to contribute to these ends and by contracting health services. Health authority roles encompass health improvement, developing HImPs, allocating funds to primary care and strengthening links with social services.

The detail of service agreements should identify shared risks (linked, where possible, to planned improvements in efficiency) and agreed contingency arrangements should these risks materialise, e.g. higher than forecast emergency admissions. Longer-term (three to five year) agreements are encouraged, building on partnership and a medium-term view of strategies and priorities, so as to minimise administration and focus on clinical issues.

Action

Ask your department's clinical director and/or business manager about local service agreements.

- How are service agreements monitored in terms of activity, costs and quality?
- How realistic are the details and requirements?
- What are the direct costs to your directorate, and how does this relate to its fully absorbed costs?
- What data were used to establish these figures?

Related reading

Appleby J (1992) *Financing Healthcare in the 1990s.* Open University Press, Buckingham.

DoH (1994) *Managing the New NHS: functions and responsibilities.* Department of Health, London.

Department of Health and Social Services (Belfast) (1998) *Fit for the Future.* The Stationery Office, London.

King's Fund (1995) *Tackling Inequalities in Health: an agenda for action.* King's Fund, London.

Leathard A (1990) *Health Care Provision: past, present and future.* Chapman & Hall, London.

NAHAT (1994) *Funding and Finance in the NHS. A Director's Guide.* National Association of Health Authorities and Trusts, Birmingham.

NAHAT (1994) *The Company Secretary in the NHS.* National Association of Health Authorities and Trusts, Birmingham.

NHSE (1998) *National Reference Costs Index.* NHS Executive, Leeds.

NHSME (1990) *NHS Trusts: a working guide.* NHS Management Executive, London.

Øvretveit J (1995) *Purchasing for Health: health services management.* Open University Press, Buckingham.

Paton C (1992) *Competition and Planning in the NHS: the danger of unplanned markets.* Chapman & Hall, London.

Scottish Office Department of Health (1997) *Designed to Care: renewing the NHS in Scotland.* The Stationery Office, London.

Scottish Office Department of Health (1999) *Towards a Healthier Scotland.* The Stationery Office, London.

Welsh Office NHS Cymru Wales (1998) *Wales: putting patients first.* The Stationery Office, London.

9

Useful information

The aim of this chapter is to provide you with information you may find useful, instructive or that you may need to know.

- Healthcare-related reports and publications.

- A glossary of health service, management, non-clinical, telemedical and computer terms.

- Useful health service acronyms.

Key reports and publications

The following list covers Acts, Circulars, Reports and Executive Letters (ELs). Although we have tried to be as comprehensive as possible, not everything is included. Some publications have been omitted as we felt they could be left out to reduce the size of the list.

Misuse of Drugs Act 1971
Covers dangerous or otherwise harmful drugs and related matters.

Health and Safety at Work etc. Act 1974
Sets out the relevant responsibilities of employers and people at work. The legal obligations ensure, as far as is reasonably possible, that employees and members of the public are not exposed to unacceptable risk as a result of the organisation's activities.

Sex Discrimination Act 1975
Makes it illegal for employers, professional bodies and trade unions to discriminate either directly or indirectly on the grounds of sex or marital status, except where marital status or a particular sex can be clearly shown to be a genuine requirement.

Medicines Labelling Regulations 1976
Rules about how medicines should be labelled.

Race Relations Act 1976
Aims to eliminate racial discrimination and to remedy individual grievances. It makes unlawful direct or indirect discrimination on the grounds of race, ethnicity or nationality in the fields of, for example, employment, education or housing.

Health and Safety (First Aid) Regulations 1981
Identifies the necessary requirements to ensure first aid can be provided in the workplace.

The Griffiths Report 1983
Report on the effective use and management of resources in the NHS set up by Sir Norman Fowler, then Secretary of State for Social Services. Consists of a short report in the form of a letter comprising only 24 pages. Ask for DHSS NHS Management Inquiry. *Griffiths Report 1983 DA(83)38*. HMSO, London.

Mental Health Act 1983 (MHA)
Provides the statutory framework under which mentally ill patients are detained and cared for in hospital. Includes patient admission (under strict guidelines) for assessment, treatment and emergency detention, and outlines the power of the courts, placing of safety orders and consent to treatment. A patient should be made aware of their admission to hospital and has a statutory right of appeal.

Data Protection Act 1984
Brings the UK into line with other Western countries in terms of the rights, duties and obligations of all persons and organisations concerned with computers and computerised data. The Act recognises the specific importance of personal data and an individual citizen's rights. The Act allows individuals right of access to information about themselves that is held on computer.

The Registered Homes Act 1984
Sets standards for the independent healthcare sector. Sets out basic standards for facilities, staffing and procedures of a registered home.

Ionising Radiations Regulations 1985
Statutory requirements to specify radiological protection measures in medical, hospital and dental work, including researchers. Replaced – *see* p. 215.

Safety and Care in the Storage, Handling and Use of Medical Cylinders on Health Authority Premises, HE1 No. 163 1987
Health equipment information guidelines issued by the Department of Health (DoH).

Guidelines for the Safe and Secure Handling of Medicines Report 1988
Also known as the Duthie (RB) Report.

Commission on the Provision of Surgical Services 1988
A report of the working party on the composition of a surgical team. Covers general surgery, orthopaedics and otolaryngology. Ask for *Commission on the Provision of Surgical Services 1988*. Royal College of Surgeons of England.

Access to Medical Reports Act 1988, Access to Health Records Act 1990 or Access to Health Records (Northern Ireland) Order 1993
Gives people right of access to their own health records and provides for the correction of inaccurate information in manually held records. Repealed by Data Protection Act 1998.

Control of Substances Hazardous to Health Regulations 1988 (COSHH)
Often referred to as the 'COSHH requirements'. Replaced – *see* p. 216.

Ionising Radiation (Protection of Persons Undergoing Medical Examination or Treatment) Regulations 1988 (SI.1988 No.778)
States that in the interest of persons (or patients) undergoing medical examinations, employers must ensure that their employees (carrying out such examinations with ionising radiation) are qualified and can produce a certificate to that effect. Employers must also keep a record of their employees' training.

The Children's Act 1989
Provides the foundation for law on children in Britain. Principles laid down include that, wherever possible, children should be cared for by their own family in a safe and protected environment, that parents still have responsibility for their children not living with them, and that both the parents and the child should be kept informed and involved in decisions about the child's future. The Act requires collaboration between agencies in the provision of services to, and the protection of, children deemed to be in need. It also places responsibilities on local authority Social Services Departments (SSD) in relation to children in need. The Act emphasises the rights of a child to make informed decisions in relation to her or his own medical care. This has major implications about consent to treatment in children.

Working for Patients 1989
This is the White Paper published in 1989, which summarises the last Conservative Government's *Strategy and Programmes for the Reforms of the NHS*. The proposals in the paper were incorporated into the *NHS and Community Care Act 1990* (NHSCCA). Ask for *Working for Patients 1989*. HMSO, London.

National Health Service and Community Care Act 1990 (NHSCCA)
Covers the establishment of NHS trusts, the financing of the practices of medical practitioners, the provision of accommodation and other welfare services by local authorities, and the establishment of the Clinical Standards Advisory Group. Also defined membership of health authorities, established the family health services

authorities (FHSA), created the internal market, NHS trusts, GP fundholders and a significant change in community-based care arrangements.

Guidelines for Change in Postgraduate and Continuing Medical Education 1990
A set of guidelines for a model of change in post-basic medical education. Ask for Gale & Grant (March 1990) *Guidelines for Change in Postgraduate and Continuing Medical Education*. British Postgraduate Medical Federation and Open University.

Heads of Agreement on Junior Doctors' Hours 1990, NHS Executive
Usually known as Junior Doctors – The New Deal.

Food Safety Act 1990
Specifies appropriate qualifications for food examiners and analysts.

HC(90)9
Health Circular covering medical and dental disciplines. Formerly HM(61)112.

Care Programme Approach for People with a Mental Illness Referred to the Specialist Psychiatric Services (HC(90)23)
Sets out the general principles of the care programme approach.

Welfare of Children and Young People in Hospital 1991
Covers all aspects of caring for children and young people in hospital.

Working Together under the Children Act (1989): a guide to arrangements for the protection of children from abuse 1991, DoH
Covers arrangements for cross-agency working on child protection policies and procedures.

The Tomlinson Report 1992
The latest of a series of reports on the future of London's health services. Ask for *The Tomlinson Report 1992*. HMSO, London.

Changing Childbirth 1992, HMSO
Guidelines for the development of maternity services.

Strategy for Information Management and Technology (IM&T) in the NHS 1992, NHS Executive
Describes a common way forward for information management and technology for all sectors of the health service in England. Information management includes both computer- and paper-based systems.

Health of the Nation: a strategy for health in England 1992, HMSO
The first attempt of a Government to produce a strategy document aimed at improving the nation's health. Produced as a White Paper it set national targets for disease prevention and health promotion in five areas to be achieved by 2000. These were coronary heart disease, cancers, mental illness, HIV/Aids and sexual health, and accidents. It identified approaches to include public policies such as food

labelling, healthy surroundings, healthy lifestyles and high quality health services. For this to be achieved, links were necessary with schools, local authorities and voluntary agencies. Ask for DHSS NHS *Health of the Nation 1992*. HMSO.

Health and Safety (Display Screen Equipment) Regulations 1992
States the minimum requirements for workstations with display screen equipment activities (in line with EC directive 901770 EEC).

Post-Registration Education and Practice for Nurses (PREP) 1992, UKCC
Introduces new legislation for the renewal of registration for nurses, midwives and health visitors and restructures all specialist post-registration education. Sets out the UKCC's requirements for education and practice following registration.

Management of Food Services and Food Hygiene in the NHS (England and Wales only), HSG(92)34
All about food handling services in the NHS.

Management of Health and Safety at Work Regulations 1992
These regulations set out broad general duties which apply to almost all work activities. Replaced – *see* p. 216.

The Cadbury Report 1992 (and Standards of Business Conduct 1993)
Outlines a code of practice that members of boards have a responsibility to the public to manage services efficiently and effectively with proper regard to corporate governance, i.e. a duty to act honestly and diligently. Concern at the time of its publication over certain managerial conduct in the NHS led to the NHSE issuing guidance entitled *Standards of Business Conduct*, as it was felt that the *Cadbury Report* was not directly transferable to the NHS.

An Introduction to the NHS in Scotland 1993
A simple explanation of the health services in Scotland, which are slightly different to England and Wales. Ask for Ham C and Haywood S *An Introduction to the NHS in Scotland*. MDG Library, Scottish Health Service Centre, Crewe Road South, Edinburgh EH4 2LF.

Tomorrow's Doctors 1993
Published in 1993 by the GMC as recommendations on undergraduate medical education. Recommends a revision of the curriculum framework, a core curriculum, special study modules and the regulation of the undergraduate course. Ask for *Recommendations on Undergraduate Medical Education 1993*. GMC.

The Calman Report 1993
Review of current specialist training and changes necessary for consistency with EC law. Also identifies areas for further review and development. The report reviews progress with the development of structured and planned training programmes, and notes the potential for the duration of specialist training to be reduced, a single training grade and introduction of Certificate of Completion of Specialist Training

(CCST). Ask for *Hospital Doctors: Training for the Future'.The Report of the Working Group on Specialist Medical Training 1993*. DoH.

Welsh Language Act 1993
Sets out provisions for the use of the Welsh language. This requires health authorities and trusts to translate into Welsh all documents, information leaflets and signs.

Mental Health Act (1983) Code of Practice 1993, HMSO
Provides guidance on the application of the Mental Health Act, section 118.

Guidance and Ethics for Occupational Physicians 1993, Faculty of Occupational Medicine

Introduction of Supervision Registers for Mentally Ill People, HSG(94)5
Covers the requirements of the supervision register. Set up to ensure continuity of care for mentally ill people, to identify those people with a severe mental illness who may be a significant risk to themselves or others and to ensure that follow-up is effective.

Guidance on the Discharge of Mentally Disordered People and their Continuing Care in the Community, HSG(94)27
Covers the discharge of people with a serious mental illness. Risk assessment illness is given extensive coverage.

Culyer Report 1994, DoH
Makes a variety of recommendations about the research and development funding systems and related topics in the NHS. An implementation plan was issued by the NHS Executive in April 1995. Ask for *Implementing Research and Development in the NHS EL(96)47*.

The Pre-Registration House Officer Experience 1994
A consensus statement from the UK Postgraduate Deans on the PRHO year. Covers standards and responsibilities, working conditions, appropriateness of clinical work, workload, education and training, educational supervision, approval of posts and living conditions. Ask for *The Pre-Registration House Officer Experience: Implementing Change 1994*. COPMED UK Conference of Postgraduate Deans.

The Wilson Report 1994
Entitled 'Being Heard', the report of a review committee on NHS complaints procedures.

Education of Sick Children, HSG(94)24
Covers aspects of providing education to children in hospital.

Ethnic Monitoring of Staff in the NHS: a programme of action, EL(94)12
A programme aimed at achieving the equitable representation of minority ethnic

groups at all levels in the NHS, reflecting the ethnic composition of the local population.

Codes of Conduct and Accountability Guidance 1994, EL(94)40, NHS Executive
Codes concerned with the conduct and account of NHS boards and their members. Standing orders should reflect the guidance that deals mainly with exchequer funds. Areas covered include annual reports, remuneration, terms of service committees, declaration of interests and register of interests.

The Patient's Charter 1991 (updated 1995)
An attempt to make public services more responsive to consumers. These were stated as basic *rights* and *expectations* as applied to the NHS. Available from *The Patient's Charter and You*, Freepost, London SE99 7XU or freephone 0800 555777. They include the following:

The Patient's Charter, (96)43
Updated in April 1995, this expanded charter sets out new rights and standards and aims to reduce waiting times. It also aims to promote the respect of dignity, privacy and patient choice.

The Patient's Charter: a charter for patients in Wales
As above but for Wales.

The Patient's Charter: services for children and young people
Sets out new rights for children and young people.

The Patient's Charter: services for children and young people in Wales
As above, again for Wales.

The Patient's Charter: mental health services
This sets out new rights for users of mental health services.

Code of Practice on Openness in the NHS 1995
Aimed at increasing access to information in the NHS. Required trusts and health authorities to make available or publish information about services, targets, standards, results, cost-effectiveness, important changes in service delivery, local health service management and who is responsible, details of public meetings, etc., and access to personal health records.

Collection of Ethnic Group Data for Admitted Patients, EL(94)77
The introduction of ethnic monitoring systems in hospitals became mandatory from April 1995.

New Deal: Plan for Action, EL(94)17
A planned approach for reducing junior doctors' hours.

The Doctors' Tale 1995

An Audit Commission report on the work of hospital doctors in England and Wales. Ask for The Audit Commission (1995) *The Doctors' Tale*. HMSO, London.

Advance Statements about Medical Treatment 1995, BMA

Gives guidance on dealing with advance directives.

Assessment of Mental Capacity: Guidance for Doctors and Lawyers 1995, BMA/The Law Society

Gives guidance on assessing a person's capacity to give valid consent.

Building Bridges: a guide to requirements for interagency working for the care and protection of severely mentally ill people 1995, DoH

Describes best practice on caring for the severely mentally ill and the importance of interagency working.

Towards Evidence-Based Practice: a clinical effectiveness initiative for Wales 1995, Welsh Office

Plans to develop evidence-based practice in Wales.

Mental Health (Patients in the Community) Act 1995

Sets out the requirements for supervised discharge for severely mentally ill people. This Act supplements Section 1 18 of the *Mental Health Act 1983*.

Children's (Northern Ireland) Order 1995

Replaces the provisions of the *Children and Young Persons Act (Northern Ireland) 1968* and amends the law relating to illegitimacy and guardianship.

Carers (Recognition and Services) Act 1995

Covers carers who are either providing, or plan to provide, a substantial amount of care on a regular basis. Under the Act, the carer is entitled to request an assessment, the results of which should be taken into account along with the needs of the patient.

Disability Discrimination Act 1995

Makes it unlawful to discriminate against disabled persons in connection with employment, the provision of goods, facilities and services for the disposal or management of premises. It makes provisions with regard to the employment of disabled persons. This Act is applicable to Great Britain.

Code of Practice on Openness in the NHS, EL(95)42

Sets out the basic principles underlying public access to information about the NHS. It complements the code of access to information which applies to the DoH/ NHS Executive and builds on the progress made by *The Patient's Charter* in this area. Requests for information should be responded to positively, except in certain circumstances, e.g. patients' records which must be kept safe and confidential.

Reporting of Injuries, Diseases and Dangerous Occurrences Regulations (RIDDOR) 1995, **HMSO**
Identifies the injuries, diseases and dangerous substances that must be reported, and the relevant authorities to which they should be reported.

Hospital Infection Control: guidance on the control of infection in hospitals, **HSG(95)10**
Contains a number of recommendations for health authorities regarding the surveillance, prevention and control of hospital infection.

Developing the Care Programme Approach – Building on Strengths 1995, **NHS Training Division**
A resource pack, developed by the NHS Training Division, enabling organisations to develop good practice around the care programme approach.

Baseline IT Security Policy in the NHS in Wales, **DGM(96)100,** *and IT Security Policy in the NHS in Wales,* **DGM(95)199**
Covers issues of security in relation to patient information.

Report of the Working Party on Alarms on Clinical Monitors 1995, **Medical Devices Agency**

The Patient's Charter Monitoring Guide: key standards, April 1996
The guide covers key Patient's Charter standards which need to be monitored nationally, and guidance on monitoring local Patient's Charter rights and standards.

Promoting Clinical Effectiveness 1996, **NHS Executive**
Describes sources of information on clinical effectiveness, suggests ways in which changes to services can be encouraged (based on well-founded information about effectiveness) and describes how changes can be assessed to see whether improvements have resulted.

Protection and Use of Patient Information, **HSG(96)18**
Guidance on the protection and use of patient information, builds on existing legislation and guidance such as the *Data Protection Act* and *Code of Practice on Openness in the NHS.*

NHS Information Management and Technology Security Manual, **HSG(96)15**
Sets out guidance on the best information-systems security practice to be adopted by the NHS.

Protection and Use of Patient Information in the NHS in Wales, **DGM(96)43**
Covers issues of confidentiality and security.

Clinical Negligence and Personal Injury Litigation, **EL(96)11**
First of a linked series of guidance notes which set out the action required by trusts and health authorities in claims handling.

NHS Complaints Procedure, **EL(96)19**
Arose out of the recommendations of the Wilson Report, 'Being Heard', and came into force on 1 April 1996.

Employment Rights Act 1996
About the employment right of employees.

The Woolf Report 1996
Lord Woolf's proposals for reform of the Clinical Negligence Scheme. Ask for *Interim Report. Access to Justice 1995*. HMSO, and *Final Report 1996*, HMSO.

A Service with Ambitions 1996
A White Paper establishing mechanisms for assessing the extent to which existing policies for professional development and training support the objectives of the NHS, encourage teamworking and create effective partnerships to ensure that educational objectives reflect changing patterns of service. It also tries to determine whether better use could be made of budgets to meet the needs of employers, and the concerns of the main professional groups.

Health and Safety (Consultation with Employees) Regulations 1996
Sets out the requirements for consultation with employees on health and safety issues.

Efficiency Scrutiny Report, Seeing the Wood, Sparing the Trees 1996, **NHS Executive**
About bureaucracy in the NHS and the 'burdens' of paperwork in NHS trusts and health authorities.

Guidance on Supervised Discharge (After-Care under Supervision) and Related Provisions, **WHC(96)11 and WOC 6196**
Covers the discharge of seriously mentally ill people in Wales.

Primary Care: delivering the future 1996
A White Paper representing a programme for action both nationally and locally, building on recent changes. It considers developing partnerships in primary care, and between primary and secondary care and local authorities. The education and training of primary care professionals, the role of research and development and the importance of clinical audit are then discussed. Proposals are made for the fairer distribution of resources and their effective use. There is also a review of workforce planning and employment opportunities, together with plans for improvements in primary care premises. The final section considers the better organisation of primary care by linking practices together, improved management support and increased use of information technology.

Health Related Behaviour: an epidemiological overview 1996
The *Health of the Nation* White Paper in 1992 emphasised the fact that an individual's health is dependent, at least in part, on their own chosen lifestyle. This paper underlines the key role of behaviour, and an understanding of health-related behaviours and the factors which influence them. Behavioural epidemiology is an important public health issue for the future. This provides an overview of the existing knowledge in this area.

NHS Waiting Times: guidelines for good administrative practice 1996
This document updates guidance issued in 1990 to waiting list managers. It gives guidance on when patients should be added to the list and the systems required to maintain it effectively. Regular reviews of the lists are necessary and the guide sets out review criteria. Procedures for the admission of patients or transfer to alternative providers are also included. It considers the role of accurate information on waiting lists in hospital management, detailing the information required by clinicians, managers and GPs.

Communication Skills: learning from patients – a training tool to help doctors reflect on their communication with patients 1996
This report presents the findings of the second stage of a College of Health project to develop a tool that will encourage doctors to think about how well they communicate with patients. Reservations were expressed about the validity of the results, but there was general agreement that the tool could be useful in training junior staff.

The New NHS Number: the key to sharing patient information 1996
The new NHS number attempts to ensure unique and unambiguous identification of each patient. The old NHS number, in 22 different formats, is prone to transcription errors and is unsuitable for computer applications. In order to overcome these shortcomings, the NHS Executive as part of its Information Management and Technology Strategy has devised the new numbering system. This booklet describes how the new NHS number is being introduced with the support of a National Implementation Team, over a two year period.

NHS Waiting Times: good practice guide 1996
Setting out the Patient's Charter guarantees and standards for waiting times as of April 1995, this guide considers the goal of delivering shorter waiting times with a booked admission date, and maintenance of local clinical priorities.

Designed to Care 1997
The NHS in Scotland White Paper. There have always been differences and variations in approach and this is reflected in this White Paper. The main

differences relate to primary care. Primary care trusts (PCTs) came into force in Scotland in April 1999.

The New NHS: modern, dependable 1997

This White Paper forms the basis for a 10-year programme to improve the NHS. It describes the replacement of the internal market by a system of integrated care, and identifies the principles underlying proposed changes. Key tasks for health authorities are defined as an assessment of health needs, including reference to HImPs, PCGs, NICE and CHI.

Animal Tissue into Humans: the report of the Advisory Group on the Ethics of Xenotransplantation 1997

Outlines the government's proposed course of action following consideration of the Advisory Group's report by government departments.

Code of Practice in the Appointment and Employment of HCHS Locum Doctors 1997

Originates from the recommendations of the Working Group on Locum Doctors, set up in December 1993. All locum appointments should comply with the Code. The main action points for trusts and others using locum agencies are listed. Details are given for the employment of locums: standards and conditions of appointment; references; health declarations; and criminal convictions.

Primary Health Care Teams Involving Patients: examples of good practice 1997

This document aims to promote awareness and stimulate thinking about appropriate ways for primary healthcare teams to involve patients.

The NHS Number: putting the NHS number to work 1997

Part of the NHSE Information Management and Technology Strategy has led to the introduction of a new NHS number that will uniquely identify each patient and allow patient information to be readily accessible but with suitable security safeguards. This booklet is intended for NHS staff and explains the benefits of the new NHS number.

A Guide to Specialist Registrar Training 1998 ('The Orange Book'), DoH

This is the official and full guide to the appointment, training and assessment of specialist registrars.

Modernising Social Services: promoting independence, improving protection, raising standards 1998

This White Paper presents the government's plans for modernising social services provision. It states the principles underlying the government's 'third way' in relation to social care.

Developing NHS Direct 1998
A study commissioned by the Operational Research Branch of the NHS Executive advocated the introduction of a nationwide 24–hour telephone advice line, which extended previous pilot studies in the use of health helplines. This report aimed to identify options for the development of such a service and provide guidance to other developments throughout the UK.

National Specialist Commissioning Advisory Group Annual Report, 1997–98
NSCAG is responsible for managing and developing highly specialised services selected for central purchasing.

Partnership in Action (new opportunities for joint working between health and social services): a discussion document 1998
As part of the White Paper *The New NHS: modern, dependable*, the government made a commitment to encourage more joint working between health and social services. This document sets out plans to make partnerships a reality so that people whose needs span both health and social services have those needs met in the most efficient and cost-effective way.

Shared Contributions, Shared Benefits: the report of the Working Group on Public Health and Primary Care 1998
This working group was set up by the DoH in 1995 with the aim of making practical proposals that would promote better co-operation between public health and primary care. *The Primary Care Act 1997* enables health authorities, primary care and public health practitioners to become involved in joint enterprises. The recent white paper *The New NHS* supports this with the development of PCGs and HAZs.

Mental Health Act 1983 – memorandum on Parts I to VI, VIII and X 1998
Designed to assist those who work with the *Mental Health Act 1983*, it offers guidance on the main provisions of the Act. The publication advises on appropriate application of the Act, and clarifies its interpretation with regard to the following areas: admission procedures; consent to treatment; court powers; mental health review tribunals; supervised discharge and aftercare; and supplementary provisions of the Act.

An Enquiry into Mentoring 1998
Supporting doctors and dentists at work – an enquiry into mentoring. A SCOPME report.

Data Protection Act 1998
Updates previous Acts and replaces Access to Medical Records Act 1990.

Public Appointments Annual Report 1998
A second annual report covering public appointments made by and on behalf of the Secretary of State for Health. The report shows those in posts at 1 March 1998 and relates to chairmen and non-executives in the following bodies: executive non-departmental public bodies (ENDPBs); advisory non-departmental public bodies (ANDPBs); health authorities; NHS trusts; special health authorities; and the Dental Practice Board. Appointments to the boards of health authorities and NHS trusts are listed by body and the NHS region in which they are located.

The New NHS Finance Function: modern, dependable. A medium-term development programme 1998
This is a response from the Finance Staff Strategy Group to the government White Paper of the same title. The identified key changes are structural, organisational, functional and external, and the support offered to help individuals manage change will be training, personal development programmes and guidance on good practice.

Composite Directory of NHS Ethnic Health Unit Projects 1998
The NHS Ethnic Health Unit (EHU) was set up in 1994 to work with ethnic minority community organisations to foster confidence in the NHS among black and minority ethnic people. This publication provides details of the 123 projects funded by the EHU between 1994 and 1997.

Smoking Kills 1998
This White Paper sets out the government's concerted plan of action to stop people smoking. It notes action already taken by the government on tobacco advertising and taxation. It goes on to present a series of measures for reducing smoking among young people, new cessation services for adults, and action on smoking among pregnant women. It then outlines proposals for abolishing tobacco advertising and promotion, altering public attitudes, preventing tobacco smuggling and supporting research. It describes further proposals for working in partnership with businesses to restrict smoking in public places, places of work and government offices, and for working with other governments at European and global levels.

General Practice Vacancies: revised selection procedures – a quick reference guide for health authorities on the revised arrangements for dealing with GP practice vacancies 1998
The NHS (Primary Care) Act 1997 set out new procedures for the selection of candidates for general practice vacancies. This document provides health authorities with a reference guide on handling vacancies.

Research and Development: towards an evidence base for health services, public health and social care – information pack 1998
Describes elements of the NHS R&D programme, the DoH's policy research programme and related research matters.

A Review of Continuing Professional Development in General Practice: a report by the Chief Medical Officer 1998
The report of a multi-disciplinary group chaired by the CMO, which set out to review the current state of continuing professional development (CPD) in general practice, and suggest directions for improvement. The group's main recommendation is that the educational process should be integrated through the creation of a practice professional development plan (PPDP).

Prescription Cost Analysis, England 1999
Prescription items dispensed in the community in England, listed alphabetically within chemical entity by therapeutic class with cost analysis and statistical data.

Getting Patients Treated: the Waiting List Action Team Handbook 1999
A handbook about reducing waiting lists and good practices relating to this in the NHS.

Quality and Performance in the NHS: clinical indicators 1999
Data were collected on six clinical quality indicators in the NHS: deaths in hospital within 30 days of surgery by method of admission; emergency admission with a hip fracture; or heart attack; emergency readmission to hospital within 28 days of discharge; returning home after treatment for a stroke within 56 days (aged 50 plus); and hip fracture within 28 days (aged 65 plus). Data are given for each area in England, classified using the 11 Office of National Statistics groups, and also by type of hospital (nine types listed). The source data was over 11 million patient episode records (1995–98).

Modernising the NHS in London 1999
A progress report on implementing the recommendations of the Turnberg report on London's health services, one year on. These include the building programme, HAZs, NHS Direct, reduced waiting lists and improved co-ordination and integration with other services.

White Paper on Modernising Government 1999
Deals with public services and their administration, the civil service, management of change and government policy in these areas.

Ionising Radiations Regulations 1999
Statutory requirements to specify radiological protection measures in medical, hospital and dental work, including researchers. Replacing *Ionising Radiations Regulations 1985*.

Control of Substances Hazardous to Health Regulations 1999
Replaces the *Control of Substances Hazardous to Health Regulations 1988*.

Management of Health and Safety at Work Regulations 1999
Broad guidelines of regulations that apply to almost all work activities. Replaces *Management of Health and Safety at Work Regulations 1992*.

Guidance on Providing Online Public Information about Local Healthcare Services 2000
In August 2000, the NHS Executive issued 10 targets associated with an additional £60 million for investment in information and IT. One relates to the online provision of accurate, standard and timely information on local healthcare services and their performance. Guidance is available on the definitive list of core information to be provided and the way in which it will be collected and published. nhs.uk will host and provide the main portal to the core information which will also be featured and accessed through NHS Direct Online.

The Vital Connection: an equalities framework for the NHS – working together for quality and equality 2000
A framework for equal opportunities in the NHS is described and a strategy is set out for putting equality aims into action. Actions to be taken by the NHS and other organisations to implement the framework are specified. Priorities for 2000–04 are listed.

Millennium Executive Team Report on Winter 1999/2000
Explains preparations taken for winter throughout the health authorities, covering resources and planning, social care, public information and immunisation programmes. The Report describes the impact of winter 1999/2000 and the consequent demand for services. A list of conclusions and recommendations are given.

UK Antimicrobial Resistance Strategy and Action Plan 2000
This document identifies surveillance, prudent antimicrobial use and infection control as the key elements to controlling antimicrobial resistance. The strategy and plan specifies eight areas for action. The aims are to minimise morbidity and mortality due to antimicrobial resistant infection and maintain the effectiveness of antimicrobial agents used in the treatment of humans and animals.

Redfern Report January 2001
Report by Michael Redfern QC on the retention and use of children's organs at the Royal Liverpool Children's Hospital (Alder Hey).

Kennedy Report 2001
Report by Prof. Ian Kennedy into children's cardiac surgery at Bristol. Completed February 2001, but published later.

Glossary of management, non-clinical and other useful terms

This is a glossary of useful terms and some definitions. Some are fairly obvious but included for the sake of completeness. The meaning may relate to a specific connection. Beware – quite often they are terms that have only a loose connection with their real meaning. You may need to check this out when you hear the expressions, but do not be surprised if the speaker is not aware of the correct meaning. A few terms are attempts that have been made to transfer manufacturing terminology to medical work.

Abduction In clinical terms a form of logical inference, commonly applied in the process of medical diagnosis. Given an observation, abduction generates all known causes. *See also* **deduction**, **induction** and **inference**.

Absenteeism Absence from work not authorised through appropriate channels.

Access rate An estimate of the availability of facilities to people living in an identified locality, irrespective of where they are treated. The measure is stated as discharges and deaths per 1000 population.

Accident Any unexpected or unforeseen occurrence, especially one that results in injury or damage.

Accident and emergency (A&E) The title given to the hospital department previously termed 'casualty'. The accident and emergency patient may be brought by ambulance or car, or may arrive on foot.

Accident report A written report of an accident. The format of the report is laid down in health and safety legislation.

Accommodation (children) Being provided with accommodation replaces the old voluntary care concept. It refers to a service that the local authority provides for the parents of children in need, and for their children. A child is not in care when they are being provided with accommodation. Nevertheless, the local authority has a number of duties towards children for whom it is providing accommodation, including the duty to discover the child's wishes regarding the provision of accommodation, and to give them proper consideration.

Accountability Being answerable for one's decisions and actions. Accountability cannot be delegated.

Added value A measure of productivity expressed in terms of the financial value of an item as a result of workforce. Often used loosely in the NHS.

Adolescents Young people in the process of moving from childhood to adulthood. Because of their age, adolescents may have special needs as patients.

Adoption Total transfer of parental responsibility from the child's natural parents to the adopters.

Advance directives A document which sets out the wishes of a patient if they are later unable to give or withhold consent for a particular treatment. This is particularly important when the patient's/user's wishes may conflict with clinical judgement.

Advocate An individual acting on behalf of, and in the interests of, patients who may feel unable to represent themselves in their contacts with a healthcare or other facility.

Affidavit Statement in writing and on oath sworn before a person who has the authority to administer it, e.g. a solicitor.

Amenity bed A bed in a single room or small NHS hospital ward for which a patient may be charged a small fixed amount for the hotel part of the cost, but not the cost of treatment, under section 12 of the 1977 NHS Act.

Analysis of expenditure by client group. Analysis of expenditure over broad groups of service related to patient care groups, e.g. services for mentally ill people, services mainly for children, and general and acute hospital and maternity services.

Functional (objective) The object for which the payment has been made – medical staff services, nursing staff services, transport services and so on.

Subjective According to the nature of the payment, e.g. salaries and wages, travel, drugs, etc.

Annual Report A report, written annually, which details progress over the last year and plans for the following year. Includes financial and activity statements.

Apology A sincere expression of regret.

Appeal (Care of Child) Appeals in care proceedings are now to be heard by the High Court or, where applicable, the Court of Appeal. All parties to the proceedings will have equal rights of appeal. On hearing an appeal, the High Court can make such orders as may be necessary to give effect to its decision.

Application In computer technology this is a synonym for a program that carries out a specific type of task. Word processors or spreadsheets are common applications available on personal computers.

Arbitration The process of settling a disagreement between two or more parties by the introduction of an external body or person with authority to make and implement an agreement.

Arden syntax A language created to encode actions within a clinical protocol into a set of situation–action rules for computer interpretation, and also to facilitate exchange between different institutions.

Area Child Protection Committee (ACPC) Based on the boundaries of the local authority, it provides a forum for developing, monitoring and reviewing the local child protection policies, and promoting effective and harmonious co-operation between the various agencies involved. Although there is some variation from area to area, each committee is made up of representatives of the key agencies, who have authority to speak and act on their agency's behalf. ACPCs issue guidelines about procedures, tackle significant issues that arise, offer advice about the conduct of cases in general, make policy and review progress on prevention, and oversee inter-agency training.

Artificial intelligence (AI) Any artefact, whether embodied solely in computer software or a physical structure like a robot, that exhibits behaviours associated with human intelligence. *See also* **Turing test**.

Artificial intelligence in medicine The application of artificial intelligence methods to solve problems in medicine, e.g. developing expert systems to assist with diagnosis or therapy planning. *See also* **artificial intelligence** and **expert systems**.

Assessment Process by which the capacities and incapacities of people who may require community care are established by social services departments, with appropriate services thereby identified.

Assessment (children) Process of gathering together and evaluating information about a child, its family and circumstances. Its purpose is to determine children's needs, in order to plan for their immediate and long-term care and decide what services and resources must be provided. Child care assessments are usually co-ordinated by social services, but depend on teamwork with other agencies (such as education and health).

Associates Salaried doctors who support principals in hard-pressed areas, such as the LIZEI area or remote parts of Scotland.

Asynchronous communication Communication between two parties when the exchange does not require both to be an active participant in the conversation at the same time, e.g. sending a letter. *See also* **synchronous communication** and **e-mail**.

Audit Originally the process by which the probity of operations and activities of an organisation was examined (internal audit) and a report on the annual accounts produced (external audit). Now used more widely, e.g. *clinical* audit evaluates the effectiveness of clinical activities; and *management* audit evaluates the effectiveness and efficiency of organisational and management arrangements. It involves the process of setting or adopting standards and measuring performance against those standards, with the aim of identifying both good and bad practice and implementing changes to achieve unmet standards.

Audit committee A committee of an NHS trust or authority board, comprising non-executive members, which ensures probity in the corporate governance of the organisation. Following *The Cadbury Report*, NHS bodies should have such a body.

Authorised person (children) In relation to care and supervision proceedings, this is a person not from the local authority who is authorised by the Secretary of State to bring proceedings under section 31 of the Act. This covers the NSPCC and its officers. Elsewhere in the Act there is a reference to persons who are authorised to carry out specified functions, e.g. to enter and inspect independent schools.

Average daily available beds The average number of staffed beds in each department in which patients are being treated, or could be treated, each day without any changes being made in facilities or staff. Beds borrowed from other departments are included.

Average length of stay The average number of days a bed is occupied by each patient.

Bayes' theorem Theorem used to calculate the relative probability of an event given the probabilities of associated events. Used to calculate the probability of a disease given the frequencies of symptoms and signs within the disease and within the normal population.

Bed bureau An administrative unit that ensures that patients needing urgent admission are directed to a hospital which will admit them.

Bed days *Available* bed days – the sum of beds available for use each day during a specified period of time. *Occupied* bed days – the sum of the number of beds occupied by patients each day during a specified period of time. This total, divided by the number of discharges and deaths during the same period, gives the average length of stay. *Vacant* bed days – the number obtained when the total of occupied bed days is subtracted from the available bed days.

Bed norm A measure of the bed requirements for a given population, expressed as number of beds per 1000 people. Bed norms may be used in several different ways: age specific, as in the case of hospital accommodation for the elderly – ten beds per 1000 aged 65 years and over; or by specialty, as in the case of orthopaedic beds – 0.35 per 1000.

Bed occupancy The number of beds occupied by patients at a particular time, usually midnight. It may be expressed as a percentage of available beds.

Bed state The number of beds, both occupied and vacant, at a particular time.

Bed turnover The average number of patients using each bed in a given period, such as a year.

Behavioural science The study of individuals and groups in a working environment. Issues may include communication, motivation, organisational structure and organisational change. The science is still being developed and relies on contributions from psychology and sociology.

Benchmarking Defined by the UK Benchmarking Centre (1993) as the continuous, systematic search for best practices, and the implementation that will lead to superior performance.

Booked case An elective admission where the date has been arranged in advance with the patient. Waiting lists should include booked cases.

British Association of Medical Managers (BAMM) Aims to 'support the provision of quality healthcare by improving and supporting the contribution of doctors in management, together with all other activities which contribute to, further, or are ancillary to this principle aim'. Contact tel: 0161 474 1141.

Budget A statement of the financial resources made available to a budget holder to provide an agreed level of service over a set period of time.

Business plan A plan setting out the goals of an organisation and identifying the resources and actions needed to achieve them. Usually prepared on an annual basis, the business plan seeks to balance planned activity with income so as to minimise financial risk.

Capital asset Land, property, plant or equipment valued at more than £5000.

Capital Asset Register A list of all the capital assets of an organisation. This contains information required to administer a capital asset replacement programme such as the purchase price, acquisition and replacement date of assets.

Capital Asset Replacement Programme A programme which uses depreciation accounting techniques to spread the cost of the replacement of capital assets.

Capital charges Since 1991, the use/ownership of capital in the NHS has incurred a cost, the capital charge. This was introduced so that NHS capital was no longer regarded as a free good or gift from the state. Capital charges consist of two elements: depreciation and interest on fixed assets. The interest rate currently applied is 6%. NHS trusts retain depreciation charges within the trust and are required to make a target rate of return equivalent to the interest rate.

Capital programme A plan over a period of time (normally five years) showing costs and starting and final dates of schemes of work to be charged to the capital allocation.

Career advice Providing information on career opportunities and training requirements.

Career counselling Discussing career options for which the individual may be most suited.

Care order (children) Order made by the court under s31 (1)(a) of the Act placing the child in the care of the designated local authority. A care order includes an interim care order except where express provision to the contrary is made.

Care plan A written statement of community care services to be provided following assessment (q.v.). The document details the care and treatment that a patient receives and identifies who delivers the care and treatment. This term covers the term 'individual plan' (*see also* **health record**).

Care Programme Approach (CPA) The individual packages of care (care programmes), developed in conjunction with social services, for all patients accepted by the specialist psychiatric services. Care programmes may range from 'minimal' single-worker assessment and monitoring for individuals with less severe mental health and social needs, to complex and multi-professional assessments and treatment.

Carer A person who regularly helps (without pay) a relative or friend with domestic, physical, emotional or personal care as a result of illness or disability. This term also incorporates friends, relatives and partners. There are thought to be six million 'informal carers'.

Case-based reasoning An approach to computer reasoning that uses knowledge from a library of similar cases, rather than by accessing a knowledge base containing more generalised knowledge, such as a set of rules. *See also* **artificial intelligence** and **expert system**.

Case conference (children) Formal meeting attended by representatives from all the agencies concerned with the child's welfare. This increasingly includes the child's parents (and the Act promotes this practice).

Casemix The mixture of clinical conditions and severity of condition encountered in a particular healthcare setting.

Cash limit A limit imposed by the government on the amount of cash a public body may spend during a given financial year. Separate cash limits may be set for revenue and capital.

Causal reasoning A form of reasoning based on following from cause to effect, in contrast to other methods in which the connection is weaker, such as probabilistic association.

Chairman A person who leads or conducts discussions. A chairman's skill and technique may be used in a one-to-one meeting or by indirect communication methods, such as the telephone.

Change agent A third party, who may be a trained behavioural scientist, and who acts as a catalyst in bringing about change by means of an organisation development programme.

Checklist A means of recording observations relating to fixed criteria; used to check compliance with agreed procedures or standards.

Child A person under the age of 18 years. There is an important exception to this in the case of an application for financial relief by a 'child' who has reached 18 years and is, or will be, receiving education or training.

Child assessment order The order requires any person who can do so to produce the child for an assessment and to comply with the terms of the order.

Child Protection Register Central record of all children in a given area for whom support is being provided via inter-agency planning. Generally, these are children considered to be at risk of abuse or neglect. The register is usually maintained and run by social service departments under the responsibility of a custodian (an experienced social worker able to provide advice to any professional making enquiries about the child). Registration for each child is reviewed every six months.

Child minder Person who looks after one or more children under the age of eight for reward, for more than two hours in any one day.

Children in need A child is in need if: (a) he or she is unlikely to achieve or maintain (or have the opportunity of achieving or maintaining) a reasonable standard of health or development without the provision for him or her of services by a local authority; or (b) his or her health or development is likely to be significantly impaired (or further impaired) without the provision for him or her of such services; or (c) he or she is disabled.

Children living away from home Children who are not being looked after by the local authority but are nevertheless living away from home, e.g. children in independent schools. The local authority has a number of duties towards such children, e.g. to take reasonably practicable steps to ensure that their welfare is being adequately safeguarded and promoted.

Clinic session A session held, and not merely scheduled, for, by or on behalf of one consultant, senior hospital medical officer or dental officer. Now extended to include sessions run by nurses and other clinical staff.

Clinical budgeting The allocation of specific budgets to consultant clinical staff who are responsible for the budget management. A part of management budgeting.

Clinical directorate A unit of management for specific clinical services. A clinical directorate is usually led by a clinical director, who is often a consultant working in that role for a number of sessions per week. They are supported by a nurse and/or business manager. The extent to which management responsibilities for budgets and staff are devolved to directorates varies.

Clinical guideline An agreed set of steps to be taken in the management of a clinical condition.

Clinical pathway *See* **clinical guideline**.

Clinical protocol *See* **clinical guideline**.

Clinical responsibilities Range of activities for which a clinician is accountable.

Closed beds Beds which have not been used (i.e. closed) for longer than one month for the purpose of redecoration or structural alterations, or because of a shortage of staff, but are scheduled to be reopened at a future date.

Code In medical terminological systems, the unique numerical identifier associated with a medical concept, which may be associated with a variety of terms, all with the same meaning. *See also* **term**.

Cognitive map A process of recording information in related groupings and intended to assist lateral thinking. *See also* **mind map**.

Cognitive science A multi-disciplinary field studying human cognitive processes, including their relationship to technologically embodied models of cognition. *See also* **artificial intelligence**.

Commissioner An organisation or individual involved in purchasing healthcare. *See also* **purchaser**.

Commissioning The process by which the health needs of the population are defined, priority healthcare needs determined, and appropriate services purchased and evaluated in order to ensure maximum health gain. It includes the wider role of influencing other agencies whose responsibilities impact on health, e.g. housing, social services and education.

Communication The two-way process of exchanging ideas, thoughts, feelings and facts.

Communication strategy A written statement of objectives for effective communication and a plan for meeting those objectives. The strategy should be consistent with the business plan.

Community care The assessment and commissioning of health and social care and treatment to patients/clients outside hospital, who have an identified physical or mental illness or disability. It is often more narrowly associated with patients being resettled from institutional care, e.g. from large psychiatric hospitals, or frail, elderly people who previously would have remained in hospital care.

Community Health Councils (CHC) 'Patient watchdog' bodies established as part of the NHS reorganisation in 1974. Their role includes assisting with complaints and visiting NHS premises. Replaced in April 2002 (*see* p. 178).

Community health services These divide into two main groups: patient care in the community – the treatment or care (outside hospital) of patients with identified physical or mental illness or disability; and services to the community – services of prevention or intervention that are provided to a population, such as immunisation, screening and health promotion.

Complainant A person who expresses dissatisfaction. They may or may not be the patient concerned.

Complaint An expression of dissatisfaction.

Complaints procedure (children) The procedure that a local authority must set up in order to hear representations regarding the provision of services under Part III of the Children's Act from a number of persons, including the child, the parents and 'such other person' as the authority considers has sufficient interest in the child's welfare to warrant his representations being considered by them.

Compliment An expression of approval or satisfaction.

Computer-based patient record *See* **electronic medical record**.

Computerised protocol Clinical guideline or protocol stored on a computer system so that it may be easily accessed or manipulated to support the delivery of care. *See also* **clinical guideline**.

Conciliation The process of a lay person assisting two parties in dispute to reach informal agreement through discussion and persuasion without any legally binding status.

Conciliatory The application of conciliation techniques particularly outside a formal conciliation process.

Concurrent jurisdiction (children) The High Court, a County Court and a Magistrates' Court (Family Proceedings Court) all have jurisdiction to hear proceedings under the Children's Act.

Connectionism The study of the theory and application of neural networks. *See also* **neural network**.

Constant prices A mechanism for comparing prices for goods and services over a number of years, which compensates for the distortion introduced by inflation.

Contact order (children) Order requiring the person with whom a child lives, or is to live, to allow the child to visit or stay with the person named in the order

Continuing education Activities which provide education and training for staff. These may be used to prepare for specialisation or career development as well as facilitating personal development.

Continuing professional development (CPD) Defined as: 'A process of lifelong learning for all individuals and teams which enables professionals to expand and fulfil their potential and which also meets the needs of patients and delivers the health and healthcare priorities of the NHS'.

Contract/Agreement A document agreed between providers and purchasers of healthcare. Details activity, financial and quality levels to be achieved.

Contract currencies Agreed units of measurement for contracting, e.g. finished consultant episodes.

Contracts The basis for agreement on the services that should be provided to patients, including specification of quality. *Block* contracts specify facilities to be provided, and may include workload agreements including patient activity targets within an agreed range. *Cost* and *volume* contracts specify the level of services required by the purchaser. Purchasers can link payment with agreed activity. Provider units will be able to match funding with workload and deploy resources more flexibly. *Cost per case* contracts cover the cost of treatment for specific patients.

Control measures Ways in which risk can be controlled, including physical controls such as locking away drugs and valuable items, and system controls such as restricting access to hazardous areas to specific staff groups.

Convenor A non-executive director of a trust, health authority or health board who decides whether or not to convene an independent panel to review a complaint against an NHS provider.

Corporate Relating to the whole of an organisation, for example the management of an organisation.

Corporate seal A seal used by organisations to certify documents used in legal transactions (such as the sale of land) so as to fulfil legal requirements.

Court welfare officer (children) Officer appointed to provide a report for the court about the child and the child's family situation and background. The court welfare officer will usually be a probation officer.

Criterion A measurable component of performance. A number of criteria need to be met to achieve the desired standard.

Cross functional team A team of people from different disciplines.

Cybernetics A name coined by Norbert Weiner in the 1950s to describe the study of feedback control systems and their application. Such systems were seen to exhibit properties associated with human intelligence and robotics, and so were an early contribution to the theory of artificial intelligence.

Cyberspace Popular term (now associated with the Internet) which describes the notional information 'space' that is created across computer networks. *See also* **virtual reality**.

Cycle time Time a patient is under treatment (in hospital). Thus, cycle time plus waiting time equals the lead time.

Database A structured repository for data, usually stored on a computer system. The existence of a regular and formal indexing structure permits rapid retrieval of individual elements of the database.

Day care (children) A person tht provides day care if they look after one or more children under the age of eight on non-domestic premises for more than two hours in any day.

Day cases Patients who have an investigation, treatment or operation, but are admitted electively and discharged on the same day.

Decision support system General term for any computer application that enhances a human's ability to make decisions.

Decision tree A method of representing knowledge that makes structured decisions in a hierarchical tree-like fashion.

Deduction A method of logical inference. Given a cause, deduction infers all logical effects that might arise as a consequence. *See also* **abduction**, **induction** and **inference**.

Designated person A person within an NHS provider, or a department of an NHS provider, who is delegated responsibility to ensure that complaints are properly resolved locally.

Direct credits The income from the sale of meals to staff, renting accommodation to staff and so on.

Direct discrimination Where someone is treated less favourably purely on grounds of marital status, sex, ethnic origin or similar criteria which do not affect the individual's ability to perform the job (*see also* **indirect discrimination**).

Disabled (children) A child is disabled if 'he or she is blind, deaf or dumb or suffers from a mental disorder of any kind or is substantially and permanently handicapped by illness, injury or congenital deformity or such other disability'.

Disclosure interview (children) Term sometimes used to indicate an interview with a child, conducted as part of the assessment for suspected sexual abuse. It could be misleading (since it implies, in some people's view, undue pressure on the child to 'disclose') and therefore the latest preferred term is 'investigative interview'.

Discrimination May be direct or indirect. For details see separate headings.

Distributed computing Term for computer systems in which data and programs are distributed and shared across different computers on a network.

Dual registered homes Homes for disabled or elderly people, registered as both a residential care home and a nursing home.

Duty to investigate (children) A local authority is under a duty to investigate in a number of situations where they have a 'reasonable cause to suspect that a child who lives, or is found, in [its] area is suffering, or is likely to suffer, significant harm'.

Education supervision order (children) Order which puts a child under the supervision of a designated local education authority.

Education welfare officer (EWO) Social work support to children in the context of their schooling. While EWOs' main focus used to be the enforcement of school attendance, today they perform a wider range of services, including seeking to ensure that children receive adequate and appropriate education and that any special needs are met, and more general liaison between local authority education and social services departments.

Educational psychologist A psychology graduate who has had teaching experience and additional vocational training. Educational psychologists perform a range of functions including assessing children's education, psychological and emotional needs, offering therapy and contributing psychological expertise to the process of assessment.

Electronic mail *See* **e-mail**.

Electronic medical record A general term describing computer-based patient record systems. It is sometimes extended to include other functions, such as order entry for medications and tests, among other common functions.

E-mail Electronic mail. A messaging system available on computer networks, providing users with personal mail boxes from which electronic messages can be sent and received.

Emergency admission A patient admitted on the same day that admission is requested.

Emergency protection order (children) That which a court can make if it is satisfied that a child is likely to suffer significant harm, or where enquiries are being made with respect to the child and they are being frustrated by the unreasonable refusal of access to the child.

Epidemiology Study of the distribution and determinants of disease in human populations.

Epistemology The philosophical study of knowledge.

Estates strategy A written statement of objectives relating to estates management and a plan for meeting those objectives. The strategy should be consistent with the business plan.

European Directive A requirement which binds an EU member state, e.g. the one designed to facilitate the free movement of doctors and the mutual recognition of their diplomas, certificates and other evidence of formal qualifications (Council Directive 93/16/EEC).

Evaluation The study of the performance of a service (or element of treatment and care) with the aim of identifying successful and problem areas of activity.

Evidence-based medicine A movement advocating the practice of medicine according to clinical guidelines, developed to reflect best practice as captured from a meta-analysis of the clinical literature. *See also* **clinical guideline**, **meta-analysis** and **protocol**.

Expert system A computer program that contains expert knowledge about a particular problem, often in the form of a set of if-then rules, that is able to solve problems at a level equivalent or greater than human experts. *See also* **artificial intelligence**.

External financing limit (EFL) A cash limit set by the NHSE on net external financing for an NHS trust. A *positive external financing limit* is set where the agreed capital spending for an NHS trust exceeds income from internally generated resources. A *zero external financing limit* is set where the agreed capital spending programme for a trust equals internally generated resources. A *negative external financing limit* is set where the agreed capital spending programme for a trust is less than internally generated resources.

Extracontractual referral (ECR) The referral of an individual for health services that was not covered in contracts that existed between the purchaser and providers of services.

Family centre Child and parents, or other person looking after a child, can attend for occupational and recreational activities, advice, guidance or counselling, and accommodation while receiving such advice, guidance or counselling.

Family Panel Panel from which magistrates who sit in the new Family Proceedings Court are selected. These magistrates will have undergone specialist training on the Children's Act.

Family Proceedings Court Court at the level of the magistrates' court to hear proceedings under the Children Act 1989. The magistrates will be selected from a new panel, known as the Family Panel, and will be specially trained.

Fieldworker (field social worker) conducts a range of social work functions in the community and in other settings (e.g. hospitals).

Financial strategy A written statement of objectives relating to financial management and a plan for meeting those objectives. The strategy should be consistent with the business plan.

Financial target (for an NHS trust) A real pre-interest return of 6% on the value of net assets, effectively a return on the average of the opening and closing assets shown in the accounts.

Finished consultant episode (FCE) An episode where the patient has completed a period of care under a consultant and is either discharged or transferred to another consultant. The total number of episodes is a common measure of overall hospital activity.

Firewall A security barrier erected between a public computer network like the Internet and a local private computer network.

Flexible training Available for doctors who have 'well-founded individual reasons' for working less than full time. The Department of Health runs two schemes to encourage flexible training for career registrars and senior registrars (PM(79)3). Flexible training for PRHOs and SHOs is available on a personal basis. In addition, a number of regions organise their own flexible training schemes.

Foster carer Provides substitute family care for children. A child looked after by a local authority can be placed with local authority foster carers.

Frequently asked questions (FAQ) Common term for information lists available on the Internet which have been compiled to newcomers on a particular subject, answering common questions that would otherwise often be asked by submitting e-mail requests to a Newsgroup.

Front line staff The employees of an NHS provider who have direct, face-to-face contact with patients and other NHS users.

Functional department Examples would include X-ray, a ward, theatre, pharmacy, pathology, a clinic or outpatients.

Functional team A team from within a single discipline.

GP fundholder A GP practice with a budget that included purchase of a range of hospital in-patient and out-patient (and certain nursing and paramedical) services. Ceased in April 1999.

Guardian ad litem (GAL) Person appointed by a court to investigate a child's circumstances and to report to the court.

Guidance (children) Authorities are required to act in accordance with the guidance issued by the Secretary of State. However, guidance does not have the full force of law but is intended as a series of statements of good practice and may be quoted or used in court proceedings.

Hawthorne effect Term used to describe changes in productivity and employee morale as a direct result of management interest in their problems. Improvements may arise before any management action. Originates from a study of the Hawthorne Works, Western Electric Co, USA (1920s).

Hazard assessment procedures The process by which the origins, frequencies, costs and effects of hazards are identified and strategies adopted to avoid or minimise their effects.

Hazards The potential to cause harm, including ill-health and injury, damage to property, plant, products or the environment, production losses or increased liabilities.

Health and safety policy A plan of action for the health, safety and wellbeing of staff, patients, residents and visitors.

Health gain The improvement of the health status of a community or population. It is sometimes described as 'adding years to life and life to years'.

Health level 7 (HL7) A healthcare-specific communication standard for data exchange between computer applications.

Healthcare professional A person qualified in a health discipline.

Health promotion Enabling individuals and communities to increase control over the determinants of health and thereby improve their health.

Health record Information about the physical or mental health of someone, which has been made by, or on behalf of, a health professional in connection with the care of that person. These must be kept for a statutory period of time after the patient is discharged from the service. Records will be held in addition to care plans.

Health Service Commissioner (HSC) The Ombudsman, appointed by Parliament to protect the rights of users of the NHS. Responsible only to Parliament.

Health service price index This index takes the NHS 'shopping basket' of goods and services (it excludes pay of employees) and weighs them according to use. The cost movement of these items is measured each month and the index updated to reflect these changes. It is used by the NHS to measure price movements and quite often to update allocations and budgets.

Health status A measure of the overall health experience of an individual or a defined population.

Hearing The process of perceiving sound or agreement to having heard a person's statement.

Herzberg's two-factor theory Herzberg maintained on the basis of research studies that in any work there are factors which satisfy and dissatisfy, but they are not necessarily opposites of each other. The latter are to do with conditions of work which he called hygiene or maintenance factors, and the former are achievement, recognition, responsibility and advancement, which he called motivators.

Heuristic A rule of thumb that describes how things are commonly understood, without resorting to deeper or more formal knowledge. *See also* **model-based reasoning**.

HMRL First of a series of hospital medical record forms. It is usually the front sheet of a patient's case notes and summarises personal, administrative and medical details. It is used for in-patients in all hospitals except those for mental illness and maternity.

Hospice NHS, voluntary or private residential premises for the provision of clinical and nursing care to residents who are terminally ill.

Hospital acquired infection An infection acquired by a patient during their stay in hospital, which is unconnected with their reason for admission.

Hospital information system (HIS) Typically used to describe hospital computer systems with functions such as patient admission and discharge, order entry for laboratory tests or medications, and billing functions. *See also* **electronic medical record**.

Hospital stay The number of days a patient stays on one hospital site during a hospital provider spell.

Hotel costs The costs of food, heating, maintenance and so on for keeping a patient in hospital, excluding all medical and treatment costs.

Human–computer interaction The study of the psychology and design principles associated with the way humans interact with computer systems.

Human–computer interface The 'view' presented by a program to its user. Often literally a visual window that allows a program to be operated, an interface could just as easily be based on the recognition and synthesis of speech or any other medium with which a human is able to sense or manipulate.

Human resource strategy A written statement of human resource objectives and a plan for meeting those objectives. The strategy should be consistent with the business plan.

Hygiene factor The element of work motivation concerned with the environment or context of job, i.e. salary, status and security, etc. To be distinguished from motivators, i.e. achievement recognition. Based on theory of Herzberg F. *See* **Herzberg**.

In care (children) Refers to a child in the care of the local authority by virtue of an order or under an interim order.

Incident An event or occurrence, especially one that leads to problems. An example of this could be an attack on one person by another within a service.

Income and expenditure reports An accountancy tool which describes and analyses the flow of funds into and out of an organisation in order to assess liquidity. Sometimes known as 'source and application of funds statements' or more commonly 'cash flow statements'.

Independent review The process of a panel of lay persons reviewing the case of a complaint where the complainant is not satisfied with the results of local resolution by an NHS provider.

Independent visitor (children) A local authority in certain sets of circumstances appoints such a visitor for a child it is looking after. The visitor appointed has the duty of 'visiting, advising and befriending the child'.

Indirect discrimination Where an unjustifiable requirement or condition is applied to the job which has a disproportionately adverse effect on one sex or group. For example, the career and life pattern of women is often different from that of men as a consequence of family responsibilities and child-bearing. Women may be less mobile than men. Another example of indirect discrimination is insisting on a conventional career path.

Individual performance review (IPR) A system of appraisal based on the setting of agreed objectives and targets between individual employees and their managers and the extent of the attainment of these targets. Normally IPR is linked to development; within the NHS it is often associated with performance-related pay for senior managers.

Induction A method of logical inference used to suggest relationships from observations. This is the process of generalisation we use to create models of the world. *See also* **abduction**, **deduction** and **inference**.

Induction programme Learning activities designed to enable newly appointed staff to function effectively in a new position.

Industrial tribunals Set up under the *Industrial Training Act 1964* they consider cases of unfair dismissal, sex discrimination and disability.

Infant mortality rate The deaths of infants under one year of age per 1000 live births.

Inference A logical conclusion drawn using one of several methods of reasoning, knowledge and data. *See also* **abduction**, **deduction** and **induction**.

Information superhighway A popular term associated with the Internet and used to describe its role in the global mass transportation of information.

Information theory Initially developed by Claude Shannon, this describes the amount of data that can be transmitted across a channel given specific encoding techniques and noise in the signal.

Informed consent The legal principle by which a patient is informed about the nature, purpose and likely effects of any treatment proposed, before being asked to consent to accepting it.

Inherent jurisdiction (children) Powers of High Court to make orders to protect a child.

Injunction Order made by the court prohibiting an act or requiring its cessation.

In-patient A patient who has gone through the full admission procedure and is occupying a bed in a hospital in-patients' department.

Inspiration trap The difficulty faced by a conciliator who can identify an obvious and sensible solution to a dispute but must ensure that the parties to the dispute reach the same conclusion without identifiable direction from the conciliator.

Integrated Services Digital Network (ISDN) A digital telephone network that is designed to provide channels for voice and data services.

Inter-agency plan (children) Plan devised jointly by the agencies concerned in a child's welfare which co-ordinates the services they provide.

Interim care order (children) Made by court, placing the child in the care of the designated local authority.

International Classification of Disease (ICD-10) Tenth edition published by the World Health Organisation for the statistical classification of morbidity and mortality. It may be used in conjunction with another classification termed Read coding.

Investigative interview (children) Preferred term for an interview conducted with a child as part of an assessment following concerns that the child may have been abused.

Investment appraisal A means of assessing whether expenditure of capital (or revenue) on a project will show a satisfactory rate of return (e.g. lower costs or higher income), either absolutely or when compared with alternative projects.

Job description Contains standard information for staff regarding conditions of service, location(s) of the post, duties of the post, accountability, education and training facilities, appraisal and the salary scale of the post. It should be available and made known to all potential applicants at the earliest possible stage and should be sent out with every application form. It contains details of accountability, responsibility, formal lines of communication, principle duties, entitlements and performance review. It is a guide for an individual in a specific position within an organisation. *See also* **person specification**.

Joint financing A sum of money taken from the health allocation and then spent on projects which are agreed by a joint consultative committee. Such monies should normally be spent on personal social service projects to reduce demands on NHS services.

Judicial review An order from the divisional court quashing a disputed decision. The divisional court cannot substitute its own decision but can merely send the matter back to the offending authority for reconsideration.

Key worker The person responsible for co-ordinating the care plan for each individual patient, for monitoring its progress and for staying in regular contact with the patient and everyone involved. A key worker may be from a variety of different professional or non-professional backgrounds.

Kipling's serving men 'I keep six honest serving men (they taught me all I know). Their names are What and Why and When and How and Where and Who'.

Knowledge acquisition Subspecialty of artificial intelligence, usually associated with developing methods for capturing human knowledge and of converting it into a form that can be used by computer. *See also* **expert system**, **heuristic** and **machine learning**.

Knowledge-based system *See* **expert system**.

Korner data Korner relates to the review of NHS information requirements by the NHS/DHSS steering group on health services information which was chaired by Edith Korner. The group recommended a minimum set of data that should be collected in all districts for management purposes.

Lay A person who is not, and preferably never has been, a professional in the field under dispute or any associated field.

Lead time Time between presentation to GP or perhaps A&E and discharge. Thus the lead time = cycle time + waiting time.

Lecture 50–55 minutes of largely uninterrupted discourse from a teacher with no discussion between students and no student activity other than listening and note taking.

Listen The process of actively hearing, accepting and understanding a verbal communication.

Local resolution The process of resolving a complaint against an NHS provider swiftly, at or very near to the point at which the issue complained about actually occurred.

Local voices initiative Encourages gathering of the views and wishes of local people as a contribution to purchasing intelligence (q.v.).

Logical To follow a sound set of rules and tests.

Looked after (children) A child is looked after when in local authority care or is being provided with accommodation by the local authority.

Mailing list A list of e-mail addresses for individuals. Used to distribute information to small groups of individuals who may, for example, have shared interests. *See also* **e-mail**.

Major incident (external) A serious external incident which requires the organisation to implement contingency plans or change or suspend some normal functions. An example would be the aftermath of a rail crash.

Major incident (internal) A serious incident occurring within the healthcare facility resulting in the changing or suspension of some normal functions or threatening of the organisation. This requires the drawing up of contingency plans. Examples of this would include the loss of electricity or telecommunications services or bomb threats.

Makaton symbols A system of symbols used to communicate with some people who have severe learning disabilities.

Management by objectives An approach to management which aims to integrate the organisation's objectives with the individual's objectives.

Management development An approach for ensuring that the organisation meets its current and future needs for effective managers. Would include succession planning, performance appraisal and training.

Manpower planning A method of ensuring that the organisation's human resources can be met now and in the future.

Matrix management A system of managing in a horizontal as well as a vertical organisation structure. Typically a person reports to two superiors, a department or line manager and a functional or project manager.

Matrix team People from different parts of the organisation and with no line authority.

Mediation The process of resolving a dispute by the intervention of an expert person who closely guides the disputing parties towards agreement.

Mentoring and co-mentoring An ancient process of learning facilitation by mutual professional support, traditionally given by a senior to a junior colleague. In co-mentoring the process of mentoring is non-hierarchical and involves co-mentees helping and supporting each other in learning.

Meta-analysis Pooled statistical analysis of results from several individual statistical analyses of different experiments, searching for statistical significance which is not possible within the smaller sample sizes of individual studies.

Mind map A process of recording information in related groupings which is intended to assist lateral thinking. *See also* **cognitive map**.

Minimum data sets A group of statistics or other information that together comprise the minimum amount of information required to inform any management process, for example for contract monitoring.

Mission statement Statement of the overall purpose of an organisation.

Model Any representation of a real object or phenomenon, or template for the creation of an object or phenomenon.

Model-based reasoning Approach to the development of expert systems that uses formally defined models of systems, in contrast to more superficial rules of thumbs. *See also* **artificial intelligence** and **heuristic**.

Monitoring The systematic process of collecting information on clinical and non-clinical performance. Monitoring may be intermittent or continuous. It may also be undertaken in relation to specific incidents of concern or to check key performance areas. It is also used in respect of selection in recording data such as sex, ethnic origin and age, etc. on applicants, short-listed candidates and appointees for retrospective review to show whether an organisation's equal opportunities policies are being carried out successfully. Monitoring also includes analysing the information and data obtained to see if there are any discrepancies in treatment/success rates of different groups, identifying the reasons and taking remedial action where appropriate. Monitoring in respect of child care is where plans for a child, and the child's safety and wellbeing, are systematically appraised on a routine basis. Its function is to oversee the child's continued welfare and enable any necessary action or change to be instigated speedily, and, at a managerial level, to ensure that proper professional standards are being maintained.

Morbidity The incidence of a particular disease or group of diseases in a given population during a specified period of time.

Mortality The number of deaths in a given population during a specified period of time.

Motivators Factors leading to job satisfaction and high employee morale. *See* Herzberg's theory of motivation.

Movement The stage in a conciliation or mediation process during which the parties modify their views and their opinions become closer to each other's.

Multi-professional A combination of several professions working towards a common aim.

Natural team For example, a boss with direct subordinates.

Neonatal death rate The deaths of infants under four weeks of age per 1000 live births. The early neonatal death rate is the deaths of infants under one week of age per 1000 live births.

Neural computing *See* **connectionism**.

Neural network Computer program or system designed to mimic some aspects of neurone connections, including summation of action potentials, refractory periods and firing thresholds.

New out-patient A patient attending for an out-patient appointment for the first time for a particular ailment. If transferred to another department, the patient is also a new out-patient on their first attendance there.

Newsgroup A bulletin board service provided on a computer network like the Internet, where messages can be sent by e-mail and be viewed by those who have an interest in the contents of a particular newsgroup. *See also* **e-mail** and **Internet**.

Non-principals A generic term for doctors who wish to practice in general practice but who do not want the financial or time commitment of becoming a principal – includes retainers, returners, assistants and associates as well as the new salaried doctor opportunities available under PCAPs.

Non-recurrent expenditure 'One-off expenditure', e.g. provision of new buildings, major alterations and major pieces of equipment. Clearly capital expenditure is non-recurrent expenditure but the purchase of minor pieces of equipment and the carrying out of maintenance work is non-recurrent, though chargeable to revenue.

Objective A clearly identifiable and quantifiable target to be achieved in the future. A specific and measurable statement which also sets out how overall aims are to be achieved.

Office of Population and Surveys (OPCS) The central government office that collects information on the entire population. Now Office for National Statistics.

Official solicitor Officer of the Supreme Court. When representing a child, the official solicitor acts as a solicitor as well as a guardian ad litem.

Ombudsman Health Service Commissioner who investigates cases of maladministration in the health service.

Open-loop control Partially automated control method in which a part of the control system is given over to humans.

Open system Computer industry term for computer hardware and software that is built to common public standards, allowing purchasers to select components from a variety of vendors and to use them together.

Opinion A belief which is held but may not be based on provable fact.

Organisation A generic term used to describe an entire organisation as opposed to the term service which is used to describe one part of the organisation (*see also* **service**). Thus a hospital, a practice or a university or medical school may all be described as organisations.

Organisation and management development strategy A written document which sets out the strategy for developing the organisational processes and management skills needed by an organisation.

Organisational chart A graphical representation of the structure of the organisation, including areas of responsibility, relationships and formal lines of communication and accountability.

Organisational development (OD) An educational strategy aimed at changing the beliefs, attitudes, values and structures within an organisation so that it can better adapt to changing requirements. The emphasis is on interventions, rather than the objective assessment of services. A systematic process of improving organisational effectiveness and adaptiveness on the basis of behavioural science knowledge.

Originating capital debt The amount owed by an NHS trust to the consolidated fund. This is equal to the value of the net assets transferred to an NHS trust when it is set up. Assets donated to the NHS since 1948 are not included.

Outcome The effect on health status of a healthcare intervention or lack of intervention. The end result of care and treatment, that is the change in health, functional ability, symptoms or situation of a person, which can be used to measure the effectiveness of care and treatment.

Out-patient A patient attending for treatment, consultation, advice and so on, but not staying in a hospital.

Output (or programme) budgets A system of analysing expenditure by reference to objectives to be met (e.g. increased level of day care; more operations) instead of under input headings such as staff and running expenses, etc.

Out-turn prices The prices prevailing when the expenditure occurs, as distinct from the estimated prices.

Paramedics Ambulance personnel with extended qualifications in providing pre-hospital care according to protocols.

Paramount principle The principle that the welfare of the child is the paramount consideration in proceedings concerning children.

Parental responsibility Defined as all the rights, duties, powers, responsibilities and authority which by law a parent of a child has in relation to the child and his property.

Part III accommodation Residential care homes provided by local authorities under Part III of the *National Assistance Act 1948*.

Parties Parties to legal proceedings under the Children's Act are entitled to attend the hearing, present their case and examine witnesses. The Act envisages that children will automatically be parties in care proceedings. Anyone with parental responsibility for the child will also be a party to such proceedings, as will the local authority. Others may be able to acquire party status.

Party A patient, carer, representative or NHS provider involved in a dispute.

Patient A person currently or previously under medical care.

Patient costing A system whereby costs are analysed in relation to specific patients or types of patient. This is the most complete analysis that can be undertaken and enables different combinations of costs to be made to fulfil any requirement. Particularly useful for evaluating proposed changes in service provision.

The Patient's Charter A list of required national standards and rights set by central government for the NHS.

Patients' council/forum/group This is a group led and determined by patients, meeting independently of staff with its own agenda and operations. There can be patient councils/fora/groups within in-patient services, day hospitals, residential or community-based services. These are different to users' groups that are separately funded and legal entities in their own right, for example charities such as the UK Advocacy Network.

Patterns of delivery The way in which services are delivered, their structure and relationship to each other. This does not relate to the content of services.

Percentage occupancy Occupied beds expressed as a percentage of the available beds during a given period.

Performance appraisal A process for assessing performance to assess training needs, job improvement plans and salary reviews, etc.

Performance indicators A standard of work that acts as a measurement of performance, for example response times to requests for work used to indicate the performance of the service. *See also* **quality indicator**.

Performance review A systematic check on the achievement of the organisation and individuals compared with set objectives.

Perinatal mortality rate Stillbirths and deaths of infants under one week of age per 1000 total births.

Permanency planning Deciding on the long-term future of children who have been moved from their families.

Personality The distinctive and identifiable characteristics of an individual human being.

Person specification Derived from the job description and outlines the qualifications, skills and experience required to perform the job. It lists what is essential and what is desirable and it should be used for shortlisting and interviewing. Person specifications should be available and made known to all those considering applying for a post so that they are aware of the criteria that will be used to judge them.

Physician's workstation A computer system designed to support the clinical tasks of doctors. *See also* **electronic medical record**.

Planning The process by which the service determines how it will achieve its aims and objectives. This includes identifying the resources which will be needed to meet those aims and objectives.

Police protection Children's Act allows police to detain a child or prevent his/her removal for up to 72 hours if they believe that the child would otherwise suffer significant harm.

Policy An operation statement of intent in a given situation.

Portfolios Personal professional development tools, aimed at encouraging reflection and self-direction in identifying training needs. They record and monitor opportunities for learning and provide tangible evidence of the outcomes. Content varies – for a job interview it will focus on practical skills, competencies and achievements, whereas for academic recognition it will reflect the ability to independently problem solve in the chosen field.

Positive action Measures by which people from particular racial groups are either encouraged to apply for jobs in which they have been under-represented or are given training to help them develop their potential and so improve their chances when competing for particular work.

Postgraduate education allowance (PGEA) GPs are eligible if they maintain a balanced programme of education and training geared towards providing the best possible care for their patients. Courses are approved (in advance) by the regional directors of postgraduate general practice education (or their staff) and can be classified in the following three areas: health promotion and prevention, disease management and service management. GPs have to show that they have attended an average of five days' training a year. Any doctor who does not take part stands to lose financially as they will not be eligible for PGEA. The structure varies and approval may be given for, e.g.:

- lunchtime lecturettes (maybe a half or quarter session)
- in-house practice meetings on specific educational topics
- week-long courses at PG centres (including at overseas resorts)
- national meetings
- reading (free) weekly medical magazines and answering MCQs on the magazine content.

Postscript In computer technology the commercial language that describes a common format for electronic documents that can be understood by printing devices and converted to paper documents or images on a screen.

Practice parameter *See* **clinical guideline**.

Preliminary hearing (children) Hearing to clarify matters in dispute, to agree evidence, and to give directions as to the timetable of the case and the disclosure of evidence.

Preventive maintenance and replacement programme A plan for the maintenance of machines to minimise the amount of time lost through breakdown by anticipating and preventing likely problems.

Primary Care Audit Group (i.e. multi-disciplinary) Groups of professionals and managers in health authorities whose remit is to encourage and facilitate the undertaking and implementation of audit in primary care – the cyclical reappraisal of structure process and outcome.

Primary care centre (PCC) Centre for out-of-hours treatment, allowed under changes to the GP contract in 1994.

Principals Doctors who have been established in general practice by the traditional route, i.e. by means of appointment to the health authorities' GMS Principal List.

Private bed (pay bed) A bed occupied by a patient who pays the whole cost of accommodation and medical and other services.

Private patient A patient who pays the full cost of all the medical and other services.

Probation officer Welfare professional employed as an officer of the court and financed jointly by the local authority and the Home Office.

Procedure The steps taken to fulfil a policy. A particular and specified way of doing something.

Professional standards Professionally agreed levels of performance.

Prohibited Steps Order (children) Order that no step which could be taken by a parent in meeting his parental responsibility for a child, and which is of a kind specified in the order, shall be taken by any person without the consent of the court.

Project 2000 The system of nurse education which places increased emphasis on student-centred and research-based learning.

Protocol The adoption by all staff of local or national guidelines to meet local requirements in a specified way. An alternative word for procedure. *See also* **clinical guideline**.

Provider A healthcare organisation, such as an NHS trust, which provides healthcare and sells its services to purchasers.

PSL GPs can apply (in accordance with paragraph 50 of the Statement of Fees and Allowances) for financial assistance in connection with a period of study leave to undertake postgraduate education, which will result in benefit to the GP, primary care (in particular) and the NHS.

Psychometric tests Standardised question and answer papers designed to measure personality.

Public dividend capital (PDC) A form of long-term government finance on which the NHS trust pays dividends to the Government. PDC has no fixed remuneration or repayment obligations, but, in the long term, the overall return on PDC is expected to be no less than on an equivalent loan.

Purchaser A healthcare body, such as a health authority or GP fundholding practice, which assesses the health needs of a defined population and buys services to meet those needs from providers.

Purchasing intelligence The knowledge purchasers need in order to make informed decisions when purchasing healthcare on behalf of their resident population. Includes demographic data, information on healthcare services, and the views of local people *(local voices)*.

Qualitative reasoning A subspecialty of artificial intelligence concerned with inference and knowledge representation when knowledge is not precisely defined, e.g. 'back of the envelope' calculations.

Quality A specified standard of performance.

Quality assurance (QA) A generic term essentially meaning that one ensures not only that the right things get done, but also that none of the wrong things are done.

Quality improvement strategy A written statement of objectives relating to quality improvement and a plan for meeting those objectives. The strategy should be consistent with the business plan.

Quality indicator A standard of service which acts as a measurement of quality, for example incidence of infection used to indicate the quality of care. *See also* **performance indicator**.

Quango A quasi-autonomous non-governmental organisation. A body with virtual statutory power.

Read coding A hierarchically arranged thesaurus of clinical condition terms which provides a numeric coding system. The system was developed by Dr Read and is cross-referenced to other national and international classifications. Developed initially for primary care medicine in the UK. Subsequently enlarged and developed to capture medical concepts in a wide variety of situations. *See also* **terminology**.

Reasoning A method of thinking. *See also* **inference**.

Recovery order (children) Order which a court can make when there is reason to believe that a child in care, who is the subject of an emergency protection order or in police protection, has been unlawfully taken or kept away from the responsible person, or has run away, is staying away from the responsible person, or is missing.

Recurrent expenditure 'Ongoing expenditure' such as salaries and wages, travelling expenses, drugs and dressings, and provisions.

Reflection The process of returning verbal or body language communication to the original perpetrator to indicate agreement and acceptance.

Refuge (children) Enables 'safe houses' to legally provide care for children who have run away from home or local authority care. A recovery order can be obtained in relation to a child who has run away to a refuge.

Regular day admission A patient who attends electively and regularly for a course of treatment and care, but does not stay in hospital through the night.

Relate A voluntary body, formerly known as the Marriage Guidance Council, which assists couples to resolve differences that threaten their relationship.

Representation The method chosen to model a process or object. For example a building may be represented as a physical scale model, drawing or photograph. *See also* **reasoning** and **syntax**.

Representations (child care) *See* **complaints procedure**.

Research and development (R&D) Searching out knowledge and evidence about the relationship between different factors in the provision of services. Research does not require action in response to findings.

Residential care homes Residential accommodation, other than group homes, providing board and lodging and personal care to the residents. Includes homes for elderly or physically disabled people.

Residential social worker (children) Provides day-to-day care, support and therapy for children living in residential settings, such as children's homes.

Resource assumptions Provisional estimates of cash resources (capital, revenue and joint finance) that may be made available over the next two to three years.

Resource management The different definitions of resource management all emphasise the involvement of doctors, nurses and other clinical staff in the continuing improvement of the quality and quantity of patient care through better use of resources and information.

Respite care Service giving family members or other carers short breaks from their caring responsibilities.

Responsibility The obligation that an individual assumes when undertaking delegated functions.

Responsible person (children) Any person who has parental responsibility for the child, and any other person which whom the child is living. With their consent, the responsible person can be required to comply with certain obligations.

Retainers Doctors appointed to practices under the Doctors Retainer Scheme who are constrained from practising full time or part time usually by virtue of domestic commitments, but who wish to keep in touch with medicine.

Returners Doctors wishing to return to clinical practice.

Revenue consequences of capital schemes (RCCS) Annual running costs of capital schemes.

Review The examination of a particular aspect of a service or care setting so that problem areas requiring corrective action can be identified.

Review (children) Local authorities have a duty to conduct regular reviews in order to monitor the progress of children they are looking after.

Review meetings The system whereby the NHSE regional offices monitor the performance of health authorities against planned objectives and set an action plan for further achievements.

Ringfencing The identification of funds to be used for a particular purpose only – usually applied to funds earmarked by central government for a particular use within the NHS or local government, e.g. the mental illness specific grant.

Risk management A systematic approach to the management of risk to reduce loss of life, financial loss, loss of staff availability, staff and patient safety, loss of availability of buildings or equipment, or loss of reputation.

Risk management strategy A written statement of objectives for the management of risk and a plan for meeting those objectives. The strategy should be consistent with the business plan.

Safe discharge of patients A procedure for the discharge of patients who require care in the community which complies with DoH guidelines.

Satisfaction survey Seeking the views of patients through responses to pre-prepared questions and carried out through interview or self-completion questionnaires.

Section 8 orders (children) The four new orders contained in the Children's Act which, to varying degrees, regulate the exercise of parental responsibility.

Secure accommodation (children) Provides for the circumstances in which a child who is being looked after by the local authority can be placed in secure accommodation. Such accommodation is provided for the purpose of restricting the liberty of the child.

Seeding The process of 'planting' all or part of an idea or plan in the mind(s) of others such that those persons produce the plan as if it were their own original thought.

Semantics The meaning associated with a set of symbols in a given language, which is determined by the syntactic structure of the symbols, as well as knowledge captured in an interpretative model. *See also* **syntax**.

Seminar A session during which prepared papers are presented to the class by one or more students.

Service The term used to describe part of an organisation, as opposed to the entire organisation. *See also* **organisation**.

Service contract A legally binding contract between an organisation and an external supplier of goods or services. The contract sets out the agreed cost and quality for a given period.

Service level agreement The term used to describe a document, agreed between organisations or services that will provide and receive a service, which sets out in detail how the service will be provided.

Significant harm (children) 'Whether harm suffered by the child is significant turns on the child's health or development; his health or development shall be compared with that which could reasonably be expected of a similar child'.

Skill mix The balance of skill, qualifications and experience of nursing and other clinical staff employed in a particular area. The process of reassessing the skill mix required is known as reprofiling.

Slippage The shortfall compared with planned spending caused by delays in the planning or execution of expenditure. Can be expressed in terms of money or time.

Social worker Generic term applying to a wide range of staff who undertake different kinds of social welfare responsibilities. *See also* **education welfare officer, fieldworker, probation officer** and **residential social worker**.

Specialty costing The analysis of costs to clinical specialties, thus enabling comparisons to be made in the same institution over time or between different institutions.

Specific issue order (children) Order giving directions for the purpose of determining a specific question which has arisen, or which may arise, in connection with any aspect of parental responsibility for a child.

Staffed allocated beds Staffed beds allocated to particular specialties including those which are available and those which are temporarily not available.

Staff Incident Reporting System A standardised system for reporting incidents and near misses. The NHSE recommends that no more than two types of forms are used for this.

Standardised mortality ratio (SMR) The number of deaths in a given year as a percentage of those expected. The expected number is a standard sex/age mortality of a reference period.

Standing financial instructions Specific instructions issued by the board of a hospital or trust to regulate conduct of the organisation, its directors, managers and agents in relation to all financial matters.

Standing orders A series of established instructions governing the manner in which business will be conducted.

Strategy A long-term plan.

Suggestion The process of putting a thought, plan or desire to another person.

Supervision order (children) Order including, except where express contrary provision is made, an interim supervision order.

Supervisor (children) Person under whose supervision the child is placed by virtue of an order.

Supraregional services Specialist services for rarer conditions provided for a population significantly larger than that of an English region. They are specially funded.

Survey The collection of views from a sample of people in order to obtain a representative picture of the views of the total population being studied.

Synchronous communication A mode of communication when two parties exchange messages across a communication channel at the same time, e.g. telephones. *See also* **asynchronous communication**.

Synergy The extent to which investment of additional resources produces a return which is proportionally greater than the sum of the resources invested. Sometimes known as the '2+2=5' effect.

Syntax The rules of grammar that define the formal structure of a language. *See also* **semantics**.

Systematised Nomenclature of Human and Veterinary Medicine (SNOMED) A commercially available general medical terminology, initially developed for the classification of pathological specimens. *See also* **terminology**.

Target allocation National share of the resources available calculated by reference to established criteria of need.

Team Any group of people who must significantly relate with each other in order to accomplish shared objectives.

Teleconsultation Clinical consultation carried out using a telemedical service. *See also* **telemedicine**.

Telemedicine The delivery of healthcare services between geographically separated individuals, using telecommunication systems, e.g. video conferencing.

Temporarily closed beds Staffed allocated beds closed for less than one month.

Term In medical terminology an agreed name for a medical condition or treatment. *See also* **code** and **terminology**.

Terminal A screen and keyboard system that provides access to a shared computer system, e.g. a mainframe or mini-computer. In contrast to computers on a modern network, terminals are not computers in their own right.

Terminology A set of standard terms used to describe clinical activities. *See also* **term**.

T group Training group, refers to training in interpersonal awareness or sensitivity, where a group of people meet in an unstructured way to discuss the interplay of the relationships between them.

Theory X A theory about motivation expounded by McGregor D, which suggests that people are lazy, selfish and unambitious, etc., and need to be treated accordingly. It contrasts with Theory Y, the optimistic view of people.

Theory Z An expression coined by Ouchi WG as a result of studying Japanese success in industry, to denote a process of organisational adaptation in which the management of the enterprise concentrates on co-ordinating people, not technology, in the pursuit of productivity.

Throughput The number of patients using each bed in a given period, such as a year. Also termed bed turnover.

Top slicing Usually used to refer to a proportional sum of money retained from budgets in a district or region to fund, e.g. region-wide initiatives, or supplement financial reserves.

Total quality management (TQM) Approach to management of organisations which aims to change organisational culture, so that continuous improvements in quality are achieved, by moving from a traditional command structure to one which encourages and empowers staff.

Training The process of modifying behaviour at work through instruction, example or practice.

Training and development strategy A written statement of objectives for the training and development of staff and a plan for meeting these objectives. The strategy should be consistent with the business plan.

Training needs analysis An approach to assessing the training or development needs of groups of employees aimed at clarifying the needs of the job and the needs of the individuals in terms of the training required.

Tribunal A court-like procedure for the resolution of disputes.

Turing test Proposed by Alan Turing, the test suggests that an artefact can be considered intelligent if its behaviour cannot be distinguished by humans from other humans in controlled circumstances. *See also* **artificial intelligence**.

Turnover interval The average number of days that beds are vacant between successive occupants.

Tutorial A discussion session, usually dealing with specified content, or a recent lecture or practical. Chaired by the teacher, it may have any number of students from one to 20 or so.

Unusual medications Medications which are currently unlicensed or being used for an unlicensed indication. Patients must be informed before they receive such medications.

Valid consent The legal principle by which a patient is informed about the nature, purpose and likely effects of any treatment proposed before being asked to consent to accepting it. *See also* **informed consent**.

Value analysis Also known as value engineering. Term used to describe an analytical approach to the function and costs of every part of a product with a view to reducing costs while retaining the functional ability.

Virement The transfer of resources from one budget heading to another. It is a means of using a planned and agreed saving in one area to finance expenditure in another area. Clear rules are needed about how virement operates so that, for instance, a budget for one-off purchases (e.g. purchase of equipment) is not spent on recurrent payments (e.g. employing staff).

Virtual reality Computer-simulated environment within which humans are able to interact in some manner that approximates interactions in the physical world.

Vital services In management terms those services that are essential to the normal operation of the organisation. Examples include electricity, water, medical gases and telecommunications.

Voice mail Computer-based telephone messaging system, capable of recording and storing messages, for later review or other processing, e.g. forwarding to other users. *See also* **e-mail**.

Waiting list The number of people awaiting admission to hospital as in-patients.

Waiting time The time that elapses between (i) the request by a general practitioner for an appointment and the attendance of the patient at the out-patients' department, or (ii) the date a patient's name is put on an in-patients' list and the date they are admitted.

Ward of court A child who, as the subject of wardship proceedings, is under the protection of the High Court. No important decision can be taken regarding the child while they are a ward of court without the consent of the wardship court.

Wardship Legal process whereby control is exercised over the child in order to protect the child and safeguard his or her welfare.

Weighted capitation Sum of money provided for each resident in a particular locality. The three main factors reflected in the formula are: age structure of the population; its morbidity; and relative cost of providing services.

Welfare checklist (children) Refers to the innovatory checklist contained in the Children's Act.

Welfare report (children) The Children's Act gives the court the power to request a report on any question in respect of a child under the Act.

Whole-time equivalents (WTEs) The total of whole-time staff, plus the whole time equivalent of part-time staff, which is obtained by dividing the hours worked in a year by part-timers, by the number of hours in the whole-time working year.

Wide area network (WAN) Computer network extending beyond a local area such as a campus or office. *See also* **local area network**.

Work in progress Waiting lists or queues waiting to be seen.

Work measurement A work study technique designed to establish the time for a qualified person to carry out a specified job to a defined level.

Work study Includes several techniques for examining work in all its contexts, in particular factors affecting economy and efficiency, with a view to making improvements.

Written agreement (children) Agreement arrived at between the local authority and the parents of children for whom it is providing services. These arrangements are part of the partnership model that is seen as good practice under the Children's Act.

Useful acronyms

The following list excludes all clinical acronyms.

AAC	Advisory Appointments Committee
A&C	Administrative and clerical
A&E	Accident and emergency
ABC	Activity-based costing
ABHI	Association of British Healthcare Industries
ABM	Activity-based management
ABPI	Association of the British Pharmaceutical Industry
AC	Audit Commission (comprises chair, deputy and 18 members all appointed by the Secretary of State from a wide range of fields)
ACAC	Area Clinical Audit Committee
ACAS	Advisory, Conciliation and Arbitration Service (set up by the UK government to assist in the resolution of disputes between employers and employees)

ACDA   Advisory Committee on Distinction Awards (consultants)

ACDP   Advisory Committee on Dangerous Pathogens

ACGT   Advisory Committee on Genetic Testing

ACHCEW   Association of Community Health Councils for England & Wales
(also **ACHC**) (local committees appoint 50%, 30% come from the voluntary sector
and the NHS Executive appoints the other members – 24 in total)

ACLS   Advanced coronary life support

ACMT   (European) Advisory Committee on Medical Training

ACOST   (Cabinet) Advisory Committee on Science and Technology

ACPC   Area Child Protection Committee

ACR   American College of Radiology

ACTR   Additional cost of teaching and research

ADC   Automatic data capture

ADH   Additional duty hours (junior doctors)

ADL   Activities of daily living

ADMS   Assistant Director of Medical Services

ADNS   Assistant Director of Nursing Services

ADP   Automatic data processing

ADR   Adverse drug reaction

ADSS   Association of Directors of Social Services

AFOM   Association of the Faculty of Occupational Medicine

AFR   Annual financial return

AGH   Advisory Group on Hepatitis

AGMETS   Advisory Group for Medical Education, Training and Staffing (an
overarching body designed to co-ordinate all issues relating to
staffing and educating doctors)

AHA   Associate of the Institute of Hospital Administrators (previously Area
Health Authority)

AHCPA   Association of Health Centre and Practice Administrators

AHHRM   Association of Healthcare Human Resource Management

AIDS	Acquired immune deficiency syndrome
AIM	Activity information mapping
	Advanced informatics in medicine
AIMS	Association for Improvements in Maternity Services
AIP	Approval in principle
ALA	Association of Local Authorities
ALAC	Artificial limb and appliance centre
ALARM	Association of Litigation and Risk Managers
ALOS	Average length of stay
AMA	Association of Metropolitan Authorities
	American Medical Association
AMP	Annual maintenance plan
AMRC	Association of Medical Research Charities
AMS	Army Medical Services
AMSPAR	Association of Medical Secretaries, Practice Administrators and Receptionists
ANDPB	Advisory non-departmental public bodies
AOP	Association of Optometrists
APH	Association for Public Health
APHI	Association of Public Health Inspectors
APLS	Advanced paediatric life support
AQH	Association for Quality in Healthcare
ARC	Arthritis and Rheumatism Council
ARSH	Association of Royal Society of Health
AS	Associate specialist
ASA	Ambulance Service Association
ASC	Action for Sick Children
ASEC	Associate Specialist Education Committee
ASH	Action on Smoking and Health

ASIT	Association of Surgeons in Training
ASSIST	Association for Information Management and Technology Staff in the NHS
ASTC	Associate Specialist Training Committee
ASW	Approved social worker
ATLS	Advanced trauma life support
ATMD	Association of Trust Medical Directors
AVG	Ambulatory visit group
AVMA	Action for Victims of Medical Accidents
AWMEG	All-Wales Management Efficiency Group
BAEM	British Association for Accident and Emergency Medicine
BAMM	British Association of Medical Managers for clinicians in, or interested in, management
BAMS	Benefits Agency Medical Service
BAOT	British Association of Occupational Therapists
BASICS	British Association of Immediate Care
BASW	British Association of Social Workers
BCS	British Computer Society
BDA	British Dental Association
	British Diabetic Association
	British Dietetic Association
BEAM	Biomedical equipment assessment and management
BGM	Board General Manager (an NHS in Scotland term)
BIM	British Institute of Management
BMA	British Medical Association
BMCIS	Building maintenance cost information system
BMIS	British Medical Informatics Society
BMJ	*British Medical Journal*
BNF	*British National Formulary*

BOPCAS	British Official Publications Current Awareness Service
BP	*British Pharmacopoeia*
BPA	British Paediatric Association
BPAS	British Pregnancy Advisory Service
BPMF	British Postgraduate Medical Federation
BPR	Business process re-engineering
BPS	British Pharmacological Society
BRCS	British Red Cross Society
BSEC	Basic Surgical Education Committee
BSI	British Standards Institution
BSR	British Society of Rheumatology
BST	Basic surgical training
BTS	British Thoracic Society
	Blood Transfusion Service
BUPA	British United Provident Association
CADO	Chief administrative dental officer
CAL	Computer assisted learning
CAMO	Chief administrative medical officer
CANO	Chief area nursing officer
CAP	College of American Pathologists
CAPO	Chief administrative pharmaceutical officer
CAS	Controls assurance statement
CASP	Critical appraisal skills programme
CASPE	Clinical Accountability Service Planning and Evaluation Specialist Healthcare Training Group
CAT	Computerised axial tomography
CATS	Credit Accumulated Transfer Scheme (a national scheme)
CBA	Cost-benefit analysis
CBS	Common basic specification

CCDC	Consultant in communicable disease control
CCE	Completed consultant episode (*see* **FCE**)
CCSC	Central Consultants and Specialists Committee (a committee of BMA)
CCST	Certificate of completion of specialist training (doctors)
CCU	Coronary care unit
	Critical care unit
CD	Clinical director
	Clinical directorate
CDC	Center for Disease Control (USA)
CDM	Chronic disease management
CDO	Chief dental officer
CDSC	Communicable Disease Surveillance Centre
CDSM	Committee on Dental and Surgical Materials
CE	Chief executive
CEA	Cost-effectiveness analysis
CEDP	Chief executive development programme
CEN	Comite Europeen de Normalisation (European Standards organisation)
CEMD	Confidential Enquiry into Maternal Deaths
CEO	Chief executive officer
CEPOD	Confidential Enquiry into Peri-operative Deaths (*see* **NCEPOD**)
CertHSM	Certificate in Health Services Management
CESDI	Confidential Enquiry into Stillbirths and Deaths in Infancy
CHC	Community Health Council (local bodies set up to protect the interests of NHS users)
CHI	Commission for Health Improvement
	Community health index
CHiQ	Centre for Health Information Quality (patient information)
CHMU	Central health monitoring unit (DoH)

CHOU	Central health outcomes unit
CHS	Child health surveillance
CHSA	Chest, Heart and Stroke Association
CIM	Capital investment manual
CIMP	Clinical information management programme
CIP(S)	Capital investment programme(s)
CIPFA	Chartered institute of Public Finance and Accountancy
CIS	Clinical information system
CISH	Confidential Inquiry into Suicide and Homicide by people with mental illness
CISP	Community information systems project
CM	Community midwife
CMB	Central Midwives Board
CMC	Central Manpower Committee (no longer exists)
CMDS	Contract/core minimum data set
CME	Continuing medical education
CMHN	Community mental handicap nurse
CMHT	Community mental health team
CMMS	Case mix management system
CMO	Chief medical officer
CMS	Community Midwifery Service
	Clinical management support
	Contract management system
CN	Charge nurse
CNM	Clinical nurse manager
CNO	Chief nursing officer
CNS	Clinical nurse specialist
	Community nursing service
	Central nervous system

CNST	Clinical Negligence Scheme for Trusts
COGPED	Committee of General Practice Education Directors
COI	Central Office of Information
COIN	Circulars on the Internet
COMA	Committee on Medical Aspects of Food Policy
COPDEND	Conference of Postgraduate Dental Deans and Directors of Education
COPMED	Conference of Postgraduate Medical Deans
COSHH	Control of Substances Hazardous to Health Legislation (1994 Regulations)
CPA	Care programme approach
	Clinical pathology accreditation
	Critical path analysis
CPAG	Capital Prioritisation Advisory Group
CPD	Continuing professional development
CPEP	Clinical practice evaluation programme
CPH	Certificate in Public Health
CPHL	Central Public Health Laboratory
CPMP	Committee for Proprietary Medical Products (EU)
CPN	Community psychiatric nurse
CPO	Chief pharmaceutical officer
CPR	Child protection register
CPSM	Council for Professions Supplementary to Medicine
CPU	Central processing unit (a microprocessor chip whose performance is a factor in the speed and performance of a PC)
CQI	Continuous quality improvement
CRAG	Clinical Research and Audit Group
CRAGPE	Committee of Regional Advisers in General Practice Education
CRC	Clinical Research Centre
CRD	Centre for Reviews and Dissemination (NHS)

CRDC	Central Research and Development Committee
CRE	Commission for Racial Equality (monitors the effects of the Race Relations Act 1976)
CRIR	Committee for Regulating Information Requirements
CSA	Child Support Agency
	Common Services Agency
CSAG	Clinical Standards Advisory Group
CSASHS	Common Services Agency for the Scottish Health Service
CSBS	Clinical Standards Board for Scotland
CSEC	Corporate Specialist Education Committee
CSM	Committee on Safety of Medicines
CSO	Central Statistical Office
CSP	Chartered Society of Physiotherapy
CSSD	Central sterile services/supplies department
CSTC	Corporate Specialist Training Committee
CT	Computerised tomography
CU	Casualties Union
CVCP	Committee of Vice Chancellors and Principals
DAP	Deans Advisory Panel
DB	Data base
DCFS	Directorate of Counter Fraud Services
DDRB	Doctors and Dentists Review Body
DEB	Dental Estimates Board
DfEE	Department for Education and Employment
DFT	Distance from target (relating to HA's financial allocation)
DGH	District general hospital
DH	Department of Health (England) (*see* **DoH**)
DHA	District Health Authority (now obsolete)
DHT	District handicap team

DI	Director of Information
DIO	District immunisation officer
DIPG	Drug Information Pharmacists Group
DIPHSM	Diploma in Health Services Management
DISP	Developing/development of information systems for purchasers
DMC	District medical committee
DMD	Drug Misuse Database
DMO	District medical officer
DMU	Directly managed unit
DN	District nurse
DNA	Did not attend
DNS	Director of nursing services
DOA	Dead on arrival
DOB	Date of birth
DoF	Director of finance
DoH	Department of Health
DPB	Dental Practice Board
DPC	Data protection commissioner
DPH	Director of public health
DPR	Data Protection Registrar
DRG	Diagnosis/diagnostic related group
DRS	Dental Reference Service
DSC	Disablement Service Centre
DSCA	Defence Secondary Care Agency
DSON	Detailed Statement of Need
DSS	Department of Social Security
	Decision support systems
DSU	Day surgery unit
DTC	Drug and Therapeutics Committee

DTI	Department of Trade and Industry
DV	Domiciliary visit (by consultant)
EAN	European article number
EBH	Evidence-based healthcare
EBM	Evidence-based medicine
EBS	Emergency Bed Service (London)
ECR	Extracontractual referral
ED	Enumeration district
EFL	External financing limit
EFMI	European Federation for Medical Informatics
EHMA	European Healthcare Management Association
EHO	Environmental health officer
EHR	Electronic health record
EIS	Executive information system
EL	Executive letter (has year and number with it)
EM	Electronic mail (e-mail)
EMAS	Employment Medical Advisory Service
EMEA	European Medicines Evaluation Agency
EMI	Elderly mentally infirm
EMR	Electronic medical record
EMS	Emergency medical services
ENB	English National Board for Nursing, Midwifery and Health Visiting
ENDPB	Executive non-departmental public bodies
ENP	Emergency nurse practitioner
ENT	Ear, nose and throat
EOC	Equal Opportunities Commission (set up under the *Sex Discrimination Act 1975* to monitor sex discrimination)
EPHR	Electronic patient health record
EPO	Emergency planning officer

EPR	Electronic patient record
EQUIP	Effectiveness and Quality in Practice Group (within DoH, chaired by CMO and CNO)
ES	Educational supervisor
ESAT	Emergency Services Action Team
ESMI	Elderly severely mentally infirm
EWO	Educational welfare officer
FBC	Full business case
FCE	Finished consultant episode (*see* **CCE**)
FCS	Financial control system
FDL	Finance directorate letter
FHom	Faculty of Homeopathy
FHS	Family Health Services (the primary healthcare providers, including GPs, dentists, pharmacists and opticians)
FHSA	(Former) Family Health Services Authority
FHSCU	Family Health Services Computer Unit
FIP	Financial information project
FIS	Financial information system
FITTA	Fixed term training appointment
FM	Facilities management
FMIP	Financial management information project
FMIS	Financial management information systems
FMP	Financial management programme
FMR	Functions and manpower review
FOM	Faculty of Occupational Medicine of Royal College of Physicians
FPA	Family Planning Association
FPHM	Faculty of Public Health Medicine
FPS	Family planning services
	Family practitioner services
FTE	Full time equivalent
FWATAG	Flexible Working and Training Advisory Group

GCC	General Chiropractic Council
GDC	General Dental Council
GDP	General dental practitioner
	Gross domestic product
GDS	General dental services
GENECIS	Generic clinical information system
GHS	General Household Survey
GLACHC	Greater London Association of Community Health Councils
GM	General manager
GMC	General Medical Council
GMP	General medical practitioner
GMS	General medical services
GMSC	General Medical Services Committee
GNP	Gross national product
GOC	General Optical Council
GOS	General ophthalmic service
GOsC	General Osteopathic Council
GPASS	General Practice Administration System Scotland
GPC	General Practitioners Committee
GPFC	General Practice Finance Corporation
GPFH	General practitioner fundholder
GPMSS	General Practice Minimum System Specification
GSM	Global System of Mobility
GTAC	Gene Therapy Advisory Committee
GUM	Genitourinary medicine
GUI	Graphical user interface
GWC	General Whitley Council
HA	Health authority
HAI	Hospital acquired infection

HAS	Health Advisory Service
HAWNHS	Health at Work in the NHS
HAZ	Health Action Zones
HB	Health Board (in Scotland)
HBG	Health benefit group
HC	Health Council
	Health circular
HCA	Hospital Caterers Association
HCAG	Hospital Consultants Advisory Group (a steering body for projects on work patterns for consultants)
HCHS	Hospital and Community Health Services (medical workforce policies)
	Hospital and Community Health Services
HE	Health education
HEA	Health Education Authority
HEBS	Health Education Board for Scotland
HEFCE	Higher Education Funding Council for England
HEFMA	Health Estates and Facilities Management Association
HELMIS	Health Management Information Service (Nuffield Institute, Leeds)
HEO	Health education officer
HES	Hospital episode statistics
	Hospital eye service
HFEA	Human Fertilisation and Embryology Authority
HFMA	Healthcare Financial Management Association
HGAC	Human Genetics Advisory Commission
HHT	Hand held terminal
HIA	Health impact assessment
HIBCC	Health Index Bar Code Council
HImP	Health Improvement Programme

HIS	Hospital information system
HISS	Hospital information and support system
HIV	Human immunodeficiency virus
HJSC	Hospital Junior Staff Committee (of BMA)
HL7	Health level 7 (a healthcare specific communication standard for data exchange between computer applications)
HLC	Healthy Living Centre
HLPI	High level performance indicator
HMR	Hospital medical record
HMO	Health maintenance organisation (USA)
HMSO	Her Majesty's Stationery Office (now **TSO**)
HO	House officer
HPR	Health process re-design
HR	Human resources
HRD–MET	Human Resources Directorate–Medical Education and Development
HRG	Healthcare Resource Group
HSAC	Health Service Advisory Committee (of HSE)
HSC	Health and Safety Commission
	Health Service Commissioner
HSDU	Hospital sterile and disinfection unit
HSE	Health and Safety Executive
HSG	Health service guidance
HSI	Health service indicators
HSJ	*Health Services Journal*
HSPI	Health Service Prices Index
HSSB	Health and Social Services Board (Northern Ireland)
HST	Higher surgical training
HSW	Health and safety at work
HSWA	*Health and Safety at Work Act 1974*

HTA	Health technology assessment
HTM	High technology medicine
HV	Health visitor
HVA	Health Visitors Association
HVHSC	The Human and Veterinary Healthcare Sectoral Consultation (bringing together interested bodies in the public and private sectors to draw up key principles concerning biotechnology and genetically modified organisms)
IAGI	Intended average gross income (of GPs) (the total money paid on average to GPs, i.e. inclusive of indirectly reimbursed expenses)
IANI	Intended average net income (of GPs) (the total money paid on average to GPs, i.e. exclusive of indirectly reimbursed expenses)
IBD	Interest bearing debt
IBNR	Incurred but not reported (clinical negligence liability)
ICD	International Classification of Disease
ICIDH	International Classification of Impairment, Activities and Participation
ICN	Infection control nurse
ICP	Integrated care pathway
ICT	Infection control team
ICU	Intensive care unit
ICWS	Integrated clinical work station
IELTS	International English Language testing service
IFM	Information for the management of healthcare
IHA	Independent Healthcare Association of 600 independent hospitals and homes
IHCD	Institute of Health and Care Development
IHE	Institute of Hospital Engineering
	International Health Exchange
IHF	International Hospital Federation
IHRIM	Institute of Health Record Information and Management

IHSM	Institute of Health Services Management
IIP	Investors in People initiative
IMA	Irish Medical Association
IMC	Information Management Centre
IMGE	was Information Management Group of NHS Executive
IMLS	Institute of Medical Laboratory Sciences
IM&T	Information management and technology
IP	In-patient
IPM	Institute of Personnel Management
IPR	Individual performance review
	Independent professional review
	Intellectual property rights
IRIS	Interactive resource information system
IRO	Industrial relations officer
ISSM	Institute of Sterile Services Management
IT	Information technology
ITU	Intensive therapy/treatment unit
JCC	Joint Consultants Committee
	Joint consultative committee
JCHMT	Joint Committee for Higher Medical Training
JCPTGP	Joint Committee on Postgraduate Training in General Practice
JDC	Junior Doctors Committee
JFC	Joint Formulary Committee
JIF	Joint Investment Fund (Scotland)
JIT	Just in time (supplies delivery)
JIP	Joint investment plan
JNC(J)	Joint Negotiating Committee on junior doctors' terms and conditions of service
JPAC	Joint Planning Advisory Committee (replaced by SWAG)

KF	King's Fund
KFOA	King's Fund Organisational Audit
KI	Key indicator (social services)
LAG	Local advisory group
LAN	Local area network
LAPIS	Locality and practice information system
LAS	London ambulance service
	Locum appointment service
LAT	Locum appointment for training
LCMG	Local communications user group
LDC	Local dental committee
LHG	Local health group (Wales)
LIG	Local implementation group
LIMS	Laboratory information management systems
LIZ	London Initiative Zone
LIZEI	London Initiative Zone Educational Incentives (a scheme of special incentives available for practitioners in Inner London until March 1998)
LMC	Local medical committee
LMWAGS	Local medical workforce advisory groups
LOS	Length of stay
LPI	Labour productivity index
LREC	Local Research Ethics Committee
LTA	Long term agreement
LURG	Local user representative group
LYS	Life year saved
MAAG	Medical Audit Advisory Group
	Multi-disciplinary Audit Advisory Group
MAC	Medical advisory committee

MADEL	Medical and dental education levy
MAF	Management accountancy framework
MAS	Minimal access surgery
MASC	Medical Academic Staff Committee
	Medical Advisors Support Centre
MBA	Master of business administration
MC	Medicines Commission
MCA	Medicines Control Agency
MCO	Managed care organisation
MDD	Medical Devices Directorate
MDDUS	Medical and Dental Defence Union of Scotland
MDG	Management development group (Scotland)
MDO	Mentally disordered offender
MDS	Minimum data set
MDU	Medical Defence Union
ME	Management executive
MEC	Management executive committee
	Management education for clinicians
MEL	Management executive letter (Scotland)
MESOL	Management education scheme by open learning
MHAC	Mental Health Act Commission
MHE	Mental health enquiry
MIDIRS	Midwife Information and Resource Service
MIMS	Monthly Index of Medical Specialties
MISG	Mental illness specific grant
MIT	Minimally invasive therapy
MIU	Minor injuries unit
MLA	Medical laboratory assistant
MLSO	Medical laboratory scientific officer

MMSAC	Medical Manpower Standing Advisory Committee (representatives from BMA, Royal Colleges, Regional Manpower committees, Medical Research Council and Council of Deans)
MOP	Mobile optical practice
MPA	Medical prescribing advisor
MPC	Medical Practices Committee
MPS	Medical Protection Society
MPT	Maximum part time
MRC	Medical Research Council
MREC	Multi-centre Research Ethics Committee
MRI	Magnetic resonance imaging
MRO	Medical records officer
MRSA	Methicillin-resistant staphylococcus aureus
MSAC	Maternity Services Advisory Committee
MSF	Manufacturing Science and Finance (technical staff trade union)
MSLC	Maternity Services Liaison Committee
MWC	Mental Welfare Commission
MWCS	Mental Welfare Commission for Scotland
MWSAC	Medical Workforce Standing Advisory Committee (working for the education committee of the GMC on appraising doctors and dentists in training for SCOPME and on general clinical training during the pre-registration year)
MWSAG	Medical Workforce Standing Advisory Group
NAAS	National Association of Air Ambulance Services
NACGP	National Association of Commissioning GPs
NACPME	National Advice Centre for Postgraduate Medical Education
NAFHP	National Association of Fundholding Practices
NAHAT	former National Association of Health Authorities and Trusts
NAHCSM	National Association of Health Care Supplies Managers
NAHSSO	National Association of Health Service Security Officers

NALHF	National Association of Leagues of Hospital Friends
NAO	National Audit Office
NATN	National Association of Theatre Nurses
	National Association of Training Nurses
NBA	National Blood Authority (England)
NBAP	National Booked Admissions Programme
NBS	National Board for Nursing, Midwifery and Health Visiting for Scotland
NBTS	National Blood Transfusion Service
NCCA	National Centre for Clinical Audit
NCCHTA	National Co-ordinating Centre for Health Technology Assessment
NCEPOD	National Confidential Enquiry into Perioperative Deaths (formerly CEPOD)
NCMO	National Case Mix Office
NCVO	National Council for Voluntary Organisations
NCVQ	National Council for Vocational Qualifications
NDPB	Non-departmental public body
NDT	National Development Team for People with Learning Disabilities
NEAT	New and emerging applications of technology
NED	Non-executive director
NeLH	National Electronic Library for Health
NET	New and emerging technologies
NF	Nuffield Foundation
NFA	No fixed address
NFAP	National Framework for Assessing Performance
NHD	Notional half day (consultants)
NHSAR	National Health Service Administrative Register
NHSCCA	NHS and Community Care Act (1990)
NHSCCC	National Health Service Centre for Coding and Classification

NHSCR	National Health Service Central Register
NHSCTA	National Health Service clinical trials adviser
NHSE	National Health Service Estates
	National Health Service Executive (England)
NHSEHU	National Health Service Ethnic Health Unit
NHSIA	National Health Service Information Authority
NHS IMC	NHS Information Centre
NHSLA	National Health Service Litigation Authority
NHSME	National Health Service Management Executive (Scotland)
NHSOE	National Health Service Overseas Enterprises
NHS(S)	National Health Service in Scotland
NHSS	National Health Service Supplies
NHST	National Health Service Trust
NHSTD	National Health Service Training Directorate/ Division
NHSTF	National Health Service Trust Federation
NHSTU	National Health Service Training Unit
NICARE	Northern Ireland Centre for Health Care Co-operation and Development
NICE	National Institute for Clinical Excellence
NIH	Nuffield Institute for Health (Leeds)
NIHSS	Nosocomial infection national surveillance scheme
NMDS	Nursing minimum data set
NMET	Non-medical education and training
NMIS	Nurse management information system
NNH	Number needed to harm
NNT	Number needed to treat
NPA	National Pharmaceutical Association
NPC	National Prescribing Centre
NPCRDC	National Primary Care Research and Development Centre

NPG	National priorities guidance
NPHT	Nuffield Provincial Hospitals Trust
NPIS	National Poisons Information Service
NPRB	Nurses Pay Review Body
NPT	Near patient testing
NRCI	National reference cost index
NRE	Non-recurring expenditure
NRPB	National Radiological Protection Board
NRR	National research register
NSC	National Screening Committee (UK)
NSCAG	National Specialist Commissioning Advisory Group
NSF	National Service Framework
NSRC	National schedule of reference costs
NSTS	NHS strategic tracing service
NSV	National supplies vocabulary
NTN	National training number
NTO	National training organisation
NTTRL	National Tissue Typing Reference Laboratory
NVQ	National vocational qualification
NWCS	NHS-wide clearing service
NWN	NHS-wide networking
O&M	Organisation and methods
OAT	Out of area treatment (the replacement for ECR)
OBC	Outline business case
OCR	Optical character recognition
OCS	Order communication system
OD	Organisational development
ODA	Overseas Development Agency
	Overseas Doctors Agency
	Operating department assistant

ODTS	Overseas Doctors Training Scheme of appropriate Royal College
OECD	Organisation for Economic Co-operation and Development
OH	Occupational health
OHE	Office of Health Economics (London)
OHS	Occupational health service
OJEC	Official Journal of the European Community
OMP	Ophthalmic medical practitioner
OP	Out-patient
OPCS	former Office of Population, Census and Surveys (system for classifying disease and treatment) Now Office for National Statistics
OPD	Out-patient department
OPM	Office of Public Management
OR	Operation research (a scientific method which uses models of a system to evaluate alternative courses of action with a view to improving decision making)
OT	Occupational therapist/therapy
OU	Open University
P&T	Professional and technical
PA	Patients Association (patient's mechanism to communicate with medical services)
PABX	Public Area Branch Exchange
PAC	Public Accounts Committee
PACS	Picture archiving and communications system
PACT	Prescription analysis and cost tabulation
PAF	Performance assessment framework
PAMs	Professions allied to medicine (physiotherapists, occupational therapists, etc.)
PARN	Professional Associations Research Network
PAS	Patient administration system
PCAG	Primary care audit group (i.e. multi-disciplinary)

PCAPs	Primary Care Act Pilots (schemes to pilot new structures of primary care delivery under the *Primary Care Act 1997*)
PCG	Primary care group
PCIP	Primary care investment plan
PCS/E	Patient Classification System/Europe
PCT	Primary care trust
PDC	Public dividend capital (a form of long-term government finance on which the NHS trust pays dividends to the government. PDC has no fixed remuneration or repayment obligations, but in the long term the overall return on PDC is expected to be no less than on an equivalent loan)
PDP	Personal development plan
PDS	Personal dental services
PEM	Prescription event monitoring
PES	Public Expenditure Survey
PESC	Public Expenditure Survey Committee
PEWP	Public Expenditure White Paper
PFI	Private finance initiative
PFC	Patient-focused care
PGD	Postgraduate dean
PGEA	Postgraduate education allowance
PGMDE	Postgraduate medical and dental education
PHA	Public Health Alliance
PHC	Primary healthcare
PHCDS	Public health common data set
PHCSG	Primary Health Care Specialist Group
PHCT	Primary healthcare team
PHL	Public health laboratory
PHLS	Public health laboratory service
PHOENIX	Primary healthcare organisations exchanging new ideas for excellence

PHPU	Public Health Policy Unit
PHSS	Personal health summary system
PI	Performance indicator
PICKUP	Professional, industrial and commercial updating
PIF	Patient information forum
PIL	Patient information leaflet
PIMS	Product information management system
PLAB	Professional Linguistic Assessment Board
PM	Project management
PMCPA	Prescription Medicines Code of Practice Authority
PMD	Performance management directorate
PMI	Private medical insurance
PMR	Physical medicine and rehabilitation
PMS	Personal medical service
	Post marketing surveillance
POISE	Procurement of information systems effectively
POM	Prescription-only medicine
POMR	Problem-oriented medical records
PoP	Point of presence (the location of the nearest node for an ISP, this is the number you dial to connect to the Internet)
POPUMET	Protection of persons undergoing medical examination (regulations)
PPA	Prescription Pricing Authority
PPC	Promoting patient choice
PPDP	Practice professional development plan
PPM	Planned preventive maintenance
PPO	Preferred provider organisation
PPP	Private Patients Plan
PPRS	Pharmaceutical price regulation scheme
PQ	Parliamentary question

PR	Public relations
PRB	Pay Review Body
PREPP	Post-registration education and preparation for practice (nurses)
PRP	Performance-related pay
PSBR	Public sector borrowing requirement
PSI	Policy Studies Institute (London)
PSL	Period of study leave (GPs can apply in accordance with paragraph 50 of the Statement of Fees and Allowances for financial assistance in connection with a period of study leave to undertake postgraduate education, which will result in benefit to the GP, primary care in particular and the NHS)
PSMs	Professions supplementary to medicine
PSNC	Pharmaceutical Services Negotiating Committee
PSNCR	Public sector net cash requirement
PSS	Personal social services
PTS	Patient transport services
PVC	Prime vendor contract
QA	Quality assurance
QALY	Quality-adjusted life year
QUANGO	Quasi autonomous non-governmental organisation
R&D	Research and development
RA	Regional advisor
RAE	Research assessment exercise
RAG	Research Allocation Group (NHS Executive)
RASP	Resource allocation and service planning
RAWP	Resource Allocation Working Party (the working party devised a method of distributing resources to health authorities equitably in relation to need, which was used from 1977–1989. The system has been superseded by weighted capitation payments)
RB	Representative Body (BMA)
RCA	Royal College of Anaesthetists

RCCS	Revenue consequences of capital schemes
	Reid clinical classification system
RCGP	Royal College of General Practitioners
RCM	Royal College Of Midwives
RCN	Royal College of Nursing
RCOG	Royal College of Obstetricians and Gynaecologists
RCOphth	Royal College of Ophthalmologists
RCP	Royal College of Physicians
RCPath	Royal College of Pathologists
RCPCH	Royal College of Paediatrics and Child Health
RCPsych	Royal College of Psychiatrists
RCR	Royal College of Radiologists
RCS	Royal College of Surgeons
RCT	Randomised controlled trial
RDRD	Regional director of research and development
RDU	Regional dialysis unit
REA	Regional education advisor
REC	Research Ethics Committee
REDG	Regional Education and Development Group
RFA	Requirements for accreditation (GP computers)
RGN	Registered general nurse
RHA	Regional health authority (now obsolete)
RHI	Regional head of information
RIPA	Royal Institute of Public Administration
RIPHH	Royal Institute of Public Health and Hygiene
RIS	Radiology Information System
RITA	Record of Individual (In-training) Training Assessment
RM	Resource management
RMC	Regional Manpower Committee (now gone)

RMI	Resource management initiative
RMN	Registered mental nurse
RMO	Resident medical officer
	Responsible medical officer
RN	Registered nurse
RNHA	Registered Nursing Home Association
RNMH	Registered nurse for the mentally handicapped
RO	NHS Executive regional office
ROCE	Return on capital employed
ROE	Regional Office for Europe (WHO)
RPSGB	Royal Pharmaceutical Society of Great Britain
RSCG	Regional specialised commissioning group
RSCN	Registered sick children's nurse
RSH	Royal Society of Health
RSI	Repetitive strain injury
RSM	Royal Society of Medicine
RSU	Regional secure unit
RTA	Road traffic accident
RTF	Regional task force
SAC	Specialist Advisory Committee (of appropriate Royal College)
SaFF	Service and financial framework
SAGNIS	Strategic advisory group for nursing information systems
SAHC	Scottish Association of Health Councils
SAMH	Scottish Association for Mental Health
SAMM	Safety assessment of marketed medicines (guidelines)
SAS	Standard accounting system
	Scottish Ambulance Service
SCBU	Special care baby unit
SCIEH	Scottish Centre for Infection and Environmental Health

SCM	Specialist in community medicine
SCODA	Standing Conference on Drug Abuse
SCOPME	Standing Committee on Postgraduate Medical and Dental Education
SCORPME	Standing Committee on Regional Postgraduate Medical Education
SCOTH	Scientific Committee on Tobacco and Health
SCPMDE	Scottish Council for Postgraduate Medical and Dental Education
SERNIP	Safety and Efficiency Register of New Interventional Procedures
SDO	Service delivery and organisation
SDP	Service delivery practice (NHS Web database)
SDU	Service delivery unit
SFA	Statement of fees and allowances
SFI	Standing financial instructions
SG	Staff grade
SGHT	Standing Group on Health Technology
SGML	Standard general mark-up language
SGUMDER	Standing Group on Undergraduate Medical and Dental Education and Research
SHA	Special health authority
SHARE	Scottish Health Authorities Revenue Equalisation
SHAS	Scottish Health Advisory Service
SHMO	Senior hospital medical officer
SHO	Senior house officer
SHRINE	Strategic human resource information network
SHTAC	Scottish Health Technology Assessment Centre
SI	Statutory instrument
SID	Sudden infant death
SIFT	Service increment for teaching
SIFTR	Service increment for teaching and research (the costs of undergraduate medical (and dental) education and research in teaching hospitals is met through SIFTR It is intended to prevent some NHS

trusts being at a disadvantage in cost terms by having to include these elements in contract prices)

SIGN	Scottish Intercollegiate Guidelines Network
SIS	Supplies information system
SLA	Service level agreement
SMAC	Standing Medical Advisory Committee
SMAS	Substance Misuse Advisory Service
SMO	Senior medical officer
SMR	Standardised mortality ratio
SNMAC	Standing Nursing and Midwifery Advisory Committee
SNOMED	Systematised nomenclature of human and veterinary medicine
SNTN	Scottish National Training Number
SODoH	Scottish Department of Health
SofS	Secretary of State
SOHHD	Scottish Office Home and Health Department
SPA	Scottish prescribing analysis
SPG	(NHS) Security Policy Group
SpR	Specialist registrar
SPS	Standard payroll system
SR	Society of Radiographers
	Senior registrar
SRD	State registered dietician
SS	Spread sheet
SSA	Standard spending assessment
SSD	Social services department
SSI	Social Services Inspectorate
STA	Specialist Training Authority of Royal Colleges
STC	Specialty Training Committee (of local postgraduate dean)
STG	Special transitional grant

STP	Short-term programme
SWAG	Specialist Workforce Advisory Group (a group focused on the number of doctors required to provide the service)
SWG	Specialty Working Group
SWOT	An analysis of strengths, weakness, opportunities and threats (usually relates to organisations but could apply equally to an individual)
T&CS	Terms and conditions of service (*see* also **TCS**)
T&O	Trauma and orthopaedics
TAG	Technical Advisory Group
TCS	Terms and conditions of service (*see* also **T&CS**)
TEC	Training and Enterprise Council
TEL	Trust executive letter
TIP	Trust implementation plan (Scotland)
TLA	Three letter abbreviation
TOD	Took own discharge
TPD	Training programme director
TQM	Total quality management
TSO	The Stationery Office (formerly HMSO)
TSSU	Theatre sterile supplies unit
TUPE	Transfer of Undertakings (Protection of Employment) Regulations 1981
UGM	Unit general manager
UKCC	United Kingdom Central Council for Nursing, Midwifery and Health Visiting
	UK Cochrane Centre
UKCHHO	United Kingdom Clearing House on Health Outcomes (Leeds)
UKTSSA	United Kingdom Transplant Support Service Authority
UKXIRA	UK Xenotransplantation Interim Regulatory Authority
ULC	Unit labour cost

ULTRA	Unrelated Live Transplant Regulatory Authority
UNISON	Public sector union for health service officers, employees, local government officers and public employees
URL	Universal resource locator
UTD	Unit training director
UTG	Unified training grade (now SpR)
UTH	University teaching hospital
VDU	Visual display unit
VFM	Value for money
VFMU	Value for money unit
VSC	Voluntary service co-ordinator
VSpR	Visiting specialist registrar
VTN	Visiting training number
VTS	Vocational training scheme (the mandatory scheme of structured experience and training in hospitals and the community for doctors planning a career in general practice)
WAHAT	Welsh Association of Health Authorities and Trusts
WAIS	Wide area information server
WAN	Wide area network
WFP	*Working for Patients*
WHCSA	Welsh Health Common Services Agency
WHDI	Welsh Health Development International
WHO	World Health Organization
WIMS	Works information management system
WIST	Women in surgical training
WO	Welsh Office
WONCA	World Organisation of National Colleges, Academies and Academic Associations of General Practitioners
WP10	Working Paper 10 (now NMET)
WP	Word processor

WPA	Western Provident Association
WTE	Whole-time equivalents (the total of whole-time staff, plus the whole-time equivalent of part-time staff, which is obtained by dividing the hours worked in a year by part-timers by the number of hours in the whole-time working year)
WTEP	Whole-time equivalent post
WTI	Waiting time initiative
YCS	Young chronic sick
YDU	Young disabled unit
ZBB	Zero base budgeting

Bibliography

Abel-Smith B (1964) *The Hospitals 1800–1948*. Heineman Educational Books, London.

Abelson J (1997) Developing high quality clinical databases. *BMJ*. **315**: 382–3.

Ackoff RL (1974) *Redesigning the Future*. Wiley, New York. *See also* Wilson RN (1959–60).

Al-Farouji M (1997) How to hit it off with your boss. *Hospital Doctor*. **7 August**: 38.

Albert T (1996) Effective writing. In: A White (ed) *Textbook of Management for Doctors*. Churchill Livingstone, London.

Albert T (2000) *Winning the Publications Game: how to get published without neglecting your patients* (2e). Radcliffe Medical Press, Oxford.

Albert T and Chadwick S (1992) How readable are practice leaflets? *BMJ*. **305**: 1266–8.

Allen I (1988) *Doctors and Their Careers*. Policy Studies Institute, London.

Allison GT (1971) *Essence of Decision: explaining the Cuban Missile Crisis*. Little, Brown and Company, Boston.

Appleby J (1992) *Financing Healthcare in the 1990s*. Open University Press, Buckingham.

Appley LA (1969) *A Management Concept*. American Management Associations. Arrow Books, New York. (First published by Hutchinson in 1967.)

Audit Commission (1992) *Homeward Bound: new course for community health*. HMSO, London.

Audit Commission. *Management Issues. Pt II. Trusting in the Future: towards an audit agenda for NHS providers*. HMSO, London.

Bailey BJ (1990) Somehow we have to stop the train wreck. *Arch Otol Head Neck Surg*. **116**: 669–700.

BAMM, BMA, IHSM and RCN (1993) *Managing Clinical Services*. Institute of Health Services Management, London.

Bark M (1997) Striking out to make a difference. *Hospital Doctor.* **7 August**: 39.

Batstone GF (1992) *Making Medical Audit Effective. Module 6: using audit for education.* Joint Centre for Medical Education, London.

Batstone GF (1990) Educational aspects of medical audit. *BMJ.* **301**: 326–8

Batstone GF and Edwards M (1994) Clinical audit: how should we proceed? *South Med J.* **10**: 1, 13–19.

Batstone G and Edwards M (1996) Multi professional audit. In: A White (ed) *Textbook of Management for Doctors.* Churchill Livingstone, London.

Baxter L, Hughes C and Tight M (1996) *How to Research.* Open University Press, Buckingham.

Beck EJ and Adam SA (1990) *The White Paper and Beyond.* Oxford University Press, Oxford.

Becker HS (1969) Problems in the publication of field studies. In: GJ McCall and JL Simmons (eds) *Issues in Participant Observation: a text and reader.* Addison-Wesley, Reading, Mass.

Beels C, Hopson B and Scally M (1992) *Assertiveness: a positive process.* Lifeskills Communications Ltd, London.

Bell D (1967) Notes on the post-industrial society. *The Public Interest.* **6** & **7** (Winter and Spring).

Bell D (1972) Labor in the post-industrial society. *Dissent.* **19.1** (Winter): 70–80.

Benatar D and Benatar SR (1998) Informed consent and research. *BMJ.* **316**: 1008.

Bennett G (1987) *The Wound and the Doctor.* Secker and Warburg, New York.

Bennis W (1992) Leadership and doctors. In: R Smith (Chair), Report of meeting of senior managers from NHS at the King's Fund College. *BMJ.* **305**: 137–8.

Beverley N (1997) NHS trusts and provision of health services. In: *NAHAT NHS Handbook 1997/98.* Section 2.6: Overview of Finances and Accountability.

Bhopal RS and Thomson R (1991) A form to help learn and teach about assessing medical audit papers. *BMJ.* **303**: 1520–2.

Billings JS (1894) *Boston Med Surg J.* **131**: 140.

Birchall E and Halett C (1996) Working together: the inter-professional relations in child protection. *Health Visitor.* **February**: 59–62.

Blanchard K, Oncken W and Burrows H (1990) *The One Minute Manager Meets the Monkey.* Collins, London.

Blau PM and Scott RW (1962) *Formal Organizations.* Chandler, San Francisco, pp.189–91.

Blumberg A (1977) A complex problem: an overly simple diagnosis. *J Appl Behav Sci.* **13(2)**: 184–9.

BMA (1990) *CCSC Guidance on Clinical Directorates*. BMA, London.

BMA (1993) *Patronage in the Medical Profession*. BMA, London.

BMA (1993) *Childcare for Doctors in the NHS*. BMA, London.

BMA (1994) *Guidelines for Good Practice in the Recruitment & Selection of Doctors*. BMA, London.

Bowden D (1996) Risk management. In: A White (ed) *Textbook of Management for Doctors*. Churchill Livingstone, London.

Boyatzis RE (1982) *The Competent Manager: a model for effective performance*. Wiley, New York.

Bradbeer AF (1954) *The Bradbeer Report. Committee of the Central Health Services Council. The Internal Administration of Hospitals*. HMSO, London.

Brody J (1992) *Managing Clinical Services: decentralisation in action*. International Team Workshop, September, London.

Bucher R and Stelling J (1969) Characteristics of professional organizations. *J Health Soc Behav*. **10**: 3–15.

Buckman R (1992) *How to Break Bad News: a guide for health care professionals*. Johns Hopkins University Press, Baltimore.

Bulstrode C and Hunt V (1996) *Educating Consultants*. Oxford University Press, Oxford.

Burrows M *et al.* (eds) (1994) *Management for Hospital Doctors*. Butterworth-Heinemann, Oxford.

Buzan T (1989) *Use Your Head*. BBC Books, London.

Cadbury A (1992) *Report of the Committee on the Financial Aspects of Corporate Governance*. Gee and Co, London.

Campbell DT and Stanley JC (1966) *Experimental and Quasi-experimental Designs for Research*. Rand McNally, Chicago.

Cang S (1978) Professionals in health and social service organizations. In: E Jaques (ed) *Health Services*. Heinemann, London.

Carnall D (1997) Career guidance for doctors. *BMJ*. **315** (5 July).

Carruthers I (1994) Total fundholding in the mainstream of the NHS. *Prim Care Manage*. **4(11)**.

Cartwright F (1977) *A Social History of Medicine*. Longman, Harlow, Essex.

Chantler C (1989) How to be a manager. *BMJ*. **298**: 1505–8.

Chantler C (1990) Management reform in a London hospital. In: N Carle (ed) *Management for Health Result*. King Edward's Hospital Fund, London.

Chantler C (1992) *Keynote address*. Conference Managing Clinical Services: Decentralisation in Action, September, London.

Chantler C (1992) *Historical background: where have clinical directorates come from and what is their purpose*. Paper prepared for Working Group of the Research Unit, Royal College of Physicians, November, London.

Chantler C (1992). Management and information. *BMJ*. **304**: 623–5.

Charlwood P (1992) *Managing Clinical Services*. Centralisation in Action. London.

Chawner J (1991) *BMA News Review*. **17(1)**: 10.

Clutterbuck D (1985) *Everyone Needs a Mentor*. IPM, London.

Clutterbuck D (2000) 'Ten core mentor competencies'. Organisations and people. *AMED*. 7(4): 29–34.

Coles C (1996) Giving talks and presentations. In: A White (ed) *Textbook of Management for Doctors*. Churchill Livingstone, London.

Cooper R (1997) *Executive IQ*. Orion Business School Books, Ayman Sawaf.

Copperfield T (1996) How to take the law into your own hands. *Hospital Doctor*. **23 May**: 41–2.

Couch JB (1994) *Health Care Quality Management for the 21 Century*. The American College of Physician Executives and American College of Medical Quality, Tampa.

Cox D (1986) *Implementing Griffiths at the District Level. A Report on Progess*. BSA Med Socio Conference, Birmingham.

Cox D (1991) Health service management – a sociological view or, Griffiths and the non-negotiated order of the hospital. In: M Bury, M Calnan and J Gabe (eds) *The Sociology of the Health Service*. Routledge, London.

Croner (2000) *Croner's Health Service Manager*. Croner Publications Ltd, Kingston upon Thames, London. Also available on disk.

Crossman R (1972) *A Politician's View of Health Service Planning*. University of Glasgow, Glasgow.

Culyer Report (1994) Research & Development Task Force. *Supporting Research & Development in the NHS*. HMSO, London.

Cummings TG and Molloy ES (1977) *Improving Productivity and the Quality of Work Life*. Praeger, New York.

Daft RL (1983) Learning the craft of organizational research. *Acad Man Rev*. **8(4)**: 539-46.

Dalton M (1964) Preconceptions and methods in men who manage. In: P Hammond (ed) *Sociologists at Work*. Basic Books, New York.

Das TH (1983) Qualitative research in organizational behaviour. *Journal of Management Studies*. **20(3)**: 301–14.

Davies R (1995) Nothing but the truth. *Hospital Doctor*. **20 July**: 27.

Davis LE and Cherns AB (eds) (1975) *The Quality of Working Life*. Volume One: *Problems, Prospects and the State of the Art*. Volume Two: *Cases and Commentary*. The Free Press, New York.

Dawe V (1992) Profession divided by its system of rewards. *Hospital Doctor*. **13 February**: 33.

Dawson B (1920) In: B Watkin (ed) (1975) *Documents on Health and Social Services 1834 to the Present Day*. Methuen and Co., London.

Day RA *How to Write and Publish a Scientific Paper*. Cambridge University Press, Cambridge.

De Bono E (1985) *De Bono's Thinking Course*. BBC Books, London.

Deerfield (1994) *Guide to Quality Management* (4e). National Association for Healthcare Quality, Glenview, Illinois.

Devlin B (1985) Second opinion. *Health and Social Services Journal*. **7 February**: 165.

Devlin B (1985) Second opinion. *Health and Social Services Journal*. **18 April**: 490.

DHSS (1972) *Management Arrangements for a Reorganised Health Service*. HMSO, London.

DHSS (1972) *Report of the Working Party on Medical Administrators*. Hunter Report. HMSO, London.

DHSS (1972) *Second Report of the Joint Working Party on the Organisation of Medical Work in Hospitals*. HMSO, London.

DHSS (1974) *Third Report of the Joint Working Party on the Organisation of Medical Work in Hospitals*. HMSO, London.

DHSS (1979) *Patients First*. HMSO, London.

DHSS (1980) *Health Service Development. Structure and management*, HC(80)8. HMSO, London.

DHSS (1980) *Patients First. A summary of comments received*. HMSO, London.

DHSS (1982) *Health Services Management. The appointment of consultants and senior registrars*, HC(82)10. HMSO, London.

DHSS (1982) *Health Service Development. Professional advisory machinery*, HC(82)1. HMSO, London.

DHSS (1982).*The National Health Service (Appointment of Consultants) Regulations 1982 (SI 1982/276), as amended in 1990 (SI 1990/1407)*. HMSO, London.

DHSS (1983) *NHS Management Inquiry*. Griffiths Report. DA(83)38. HMSO, London.

DHSS (1986) *Health Services Management: resource management (management budgeting) in health authorities*, HN(86)34. HMSO, London.

DHSS (1988) *The New Hospital Staff Grade*, HC(88)58. HMSO, London.

DHSS (1989) *Working for Patients*. HMSO, London.

DHSS (1989) *Health Services Management. Appointment procedure for registrars*, EL(89)MB/68. HMSO, London.

DHSS (1989) *Working Together: under the Children Act*. HMSO, London.

DHSS (1990) *Health Services Management. The appointment of consultants and directors of public health*, HC(90)19. HMSO, London.

DHSS (1990) *GP Practice Vacancies: revised selection procedures*, HN(90)26. HMSO, London.

DHSS (1990) *Informed Consent*, HC(90)22. HMSO, London.

Diesing P (1972) *Patterns of Discovery in the Social Sciences*. Routledge & Kegan Paul, London.

Disken S, Dixon M and Halpern S *et al* (1990) *Models of Clinical Management*. Institute of Health Services Management, London.

Dixon M (1991). In: R Hey (1991) Code of conduct needed to keep managers in line. *Hospital Doctor*. **5 December**: 28.

Dixon M (1991) *Medical Audit Primer*. Healthcare Quality Quest, Romsey.

DoH (1989) *The Children's Act 1989*. Department of Health, London.

DoH (1989) *Working for Patients*. Working Paper 6. Command 555. HMSO, London.

DoH (1989) *Working for Patients*. Working Paper 2. Funding and Contracts for Hospital Services. Department of Health, London.

DoH (1991) *The Patient's Charter*. Department of Health Publications, PO Box 410.

DoH (1992) *NHS Guidelines – patients who die in hospital*, HSG(92). Department of Health, London.

DoH (1993) *Clinical Audit: meeting and improving standards in healthcare*. Department of Health, London.

DoH (1994) *Managing the New NHS: functions and responsibilities*. Department of Health, London.

DoH (1994) *Research and Development in the New NHS*. Department of Health, London.

DoH (1996) *Promoting Clinical Effectiveness*. Department of Health, London.

DoH (1997/98) *Priorities and planning guidance for the NHS 1997/98*. Department of Health, London.

DoH (1998) *A Guide to Specialist Registrar Training*. Section 6: Appointment to the grade. 3753 1P 48K March (03). Department of Health, London.

Donabedian A (1980) *Definition of Quality and Approaches to its Assessment*. Health Administration Press, Ann Arbor, Michigan.

Doyal L (1998) Informed consent – a response to recent correspondence. *BMJ*. **316**: 1000–1.

Drexler A, Yenney SL and Hohman J (1977) OD an ongoing program. *Hospitals*. **16 February**: 89–92.

Drife JO (1985) Be interviewed. In: *How To Do It*. Vol. 1 (2e). BMJ, London.

Drucker PF (1968) *The Practice of Management*. Pan Books, London.

Druker PF (1977) *Management. Tasks, responsibilities, practices*. Pan Business Management, London.

Druker PF (1990) *Managing the Non-Profit Organization*. Harper Collins. New York.

Drucker PF (1992) In: J Stephany (1992) *The Role of Consultant Physicians in Clinical Directorates*. Prepared for Working Group of Research Unit of Royal College of Physicians, London.

Dyregrow A (1991) *Grief in Childhood: a handbook for adults*. Jessica Kingsley, London.

Earl MJ and Skyrme DJ (undated) *Hybrid Managers. What do we know about them?* Research Paper. Oxford Institute of Information Management, Oxford.

Eddy DM (1990) Clinical decision making: from theory to practice. The challenge. *JAMA*. **263**: 287–90.

Eden C, Jones S and Sims DPB (1983). *Messing About in Problems*. Pergamon, Oxford.

Eggert M (1992) *The Perfect Interview – all you need to get it right first time*. Century, London.

EL(91)72 (1991) *Framework of Audit for Nursing Services: guidance document*. NHS Management Executive.

EL(95) *Priorities and Planning Guidance for the NHS, 1996/7*.

EL(95)37 *Acting on Complaints*.

EL(95)42 *Code of Practice on Openness in the National Health Service (England)*.

EL(95)46 *Supporting R & D in the NHS: implementation plan*.

EL(95)60 *Guidance on Implementation of Code of Practice on Openness*.

EL(95)100 *Declaration of the NHS Audit and Costs Associated with Research & Development: initial guidance*.

EL(95)121 *Implementation of New Complaints Procedure – interim guidance*.

EL(95)127 *Supporting R & D in the NHS: a declaration of NHS activities and costs associated with R & D; guidance on costing and making the declaration*.

EL(96)5 *Acting on Complaints: training for local resolution*.

EL(96)19 *Implementation of New Complaints Procedure: final guidance*.

Elliott J (1978) *Health Services*. Heinemann, London.

Ellis N and Stanton T (eds) (1994) *Making Sense of Partnerships*. Radcliffe Medical Press, Oxford.

Engel GV (1969) The effect of bureaucracy on the professional autonomy of the physician. *Journal of Health and Social Behaviour*. **10**: 30–41.

Enthoven AC (1985) *Reflections on the Management of the National Health Service*. Nuffield Provincial Hospitals Trust, London.

EOC (1990) *Equality Management; women's employment in the NHS*. A Survey Report by the Equal Opportunities Commission.

Esmail A and Everington S (1993) Racial discrimination against doctors from ethnic minorities. *BMJ*. **306**: 691–2.

Etzioni A (1968) *The Active Society*. Free Press, New York.

Etzioni A (1969) *The Semi-Professions and their Organisation*. Free Press, London.

Evans H (1972) *Newsman's English*. Heinemann, London.

Evans N (1991) There must be a better way. *BMJ*. **303**: 1483.

Fallowfield I (1993) Giving sad and bad news. *Lancet*. **341**: 476–8.

Faulkner A (1998) *When the News is Bad: a guide for health professionals*. Stanley Thornes, Cheltenham.

Fielding GH (1929) *An Introduction to the History of Medicine* (4e). WB Saunders Co., Philadelphia.

Fisher D (1980) A review of organization development. *Journal of Nursing Administration*. **October**: 31–6.

Fitzgerald L and Sturt J (1992) Clinicians into management. On the change agenda or not? *Health Services Management Research*. **5**(2 July): 137-46.

Fitzpatrick R (1996) Telling patients there is nothing wrong. *BMJ*. **313**: 311.

Fitzsimmons P and White T (1997) Crossing boundaries: communication between professional groups. *Journal of Management in Medicine*. **11(2)**: 96–101.

Flesch R (1951) *The Art of Readable Writing*. Collier Books. Macmillan, London.

Fontana D (1989) *Managing Stress*. British Psychological Society/Routledge, London.

Foot M (1962) *Aneurin Bevan: a biography*. MacGibbon and Kee, London.

Ford J (1975) *Paradigms and fairy tales* (2 vols). Routledge & Kegan Paul, London.

Francis D and Woodcock M (1996) *The New Unblocked Manager*. Gower, London.

Frater A and Spiby J (1990) *Measured Progress – Medical Audit for Physicians. A manual of theory and practice*. North West Thames Regional Health Authority.

Freidson E (1970) *The Profession of Medicine: a study of the sociology of applied knowledge*. Dodd Mead, New York.

Freidson E (1970) *Professional Dominance: The social structure of medical care*. Aldine Publishing Co., Chicago.

French S (1993) *Practical Research. A guide for therapists*. Butterworth Heinmann, London.

Friedlander F (1976) OD reaches adolescence: an exploration of its underlying values. *Journal of Applied Behavioural Science.* **12**: 1.

Friedman E (1991) The uninsured. *JAMA.* **265(19)**: 2491–5.

Galbraith S (1991) Chartered Institute of Public Finance and Accountancy Conference. *Health Service Journal.* **20 June**.

Gale R and Grant J (1990) *Managing Change in a Medical Context. Guidelines for Action.* The Joint Centre for Educational Research and Development in Medicine, London.

Gans H (1967) *The Levittowners.* Pantheon, New York.

Gatrell J and White A (1995) *Medical Student to Medical Director, A Development Strategy for Doctors.* NHS Training Division, Bristol.

Gatrell J and White A (1996) Interviews and interviewing skills. In: A White (ed) *Textbook of Management for Doctors.* Churchill Livingstone, London.

Gatrell J and White A (1996) Doctors and management – the development dilemma. *Journal of Management in Medicine.* **10(2)**.

Gatrell J and White A (1997) Appointing specialist registrars. *Clinician in Management.* **6(1)**.

Gatrell J and White A (1997) Selecting doctors – making the most of the panel interview. Medical Interface. *Journal of Disease Management.* **February**: 21–3.

Gatrell J and White T (2000) *Medical Appraisal, Selection and Revalidation.* Royal Society of Medicine, London.

Georgopoulos BS (1972) *Organization Research on Health Care Institutions.* Institute for Social Research. University of Michigan, Ann Arbor, Michigan.

Gibb F (1995) Please call the witness. *The Times.* Tuesday 12 September.

Gilley J (ed) (1994) *Women in General Practice.* BMA, London.

Gillon R (1985) Telling the truth and medical ethics. *BMJ.* **291**: 1556–7.

Gillon R (1992) *Philosophical Medical Ethics.* John Wiley, Chichester.

Gioia DA, Donnellon A and Sims HP (1989) Communication and cognition in appraisal: a tale of two paradigms. *Organization Studies.* **10(4)**: 503–30.

Glaser BG (1978) *Theoretical Sensitivity.* Sociology Press, San Francisco.

Glaser BG and Strauss AL (1967) *The Discovery of Grounded Theory: strategies for qualitative research.* Aldine, New York.

Gluckman M and Devons E (eds) (1964) *Closed Systems and Open Minds.* Aldine, Chicago.

GMC (1997) *The New Doctor.* General Medical Council, London.

Golembiewski RT (1969) Organization development in public agencies: perspectives on theory and practice. *Public Administration Review.* **29** (July/August): 367–77.

Goodare H (1998) Studies that do not have informed consent from participants should not be published. *BMJ*. **316**: 1004–5.

Goode WJ (1969) The theoretical limits of professionalisation. In: A Etzioni (ed) *Semi-professions and their Organisation*. Free Press, New York.

Goodman NW and Edwards MB (1991) *Medical Writing: a prescription for clarity*. Cambridge University Press, Cambridge.

Goss MEW (1961) Influence and authority among physicians in an out-patient clinic. *American Sociological Review*. **26**: 39–50.

Gowers E (1986) *The Complete Plain Words* (3e). Revised by Sidney Greenbaum and Janet Whitcut. HMSO, London.

Greenhalgh T (1997) *BMJ*. **315**: 80.

Greenhalgh T (1997) Getting your bearings. *BMJ*. **315**: 243–6.

Greenhalgh T (1997) Papers that tell you what things cost. *BMJ*. **315** (6 September).

Greenhalgh T (1997) Statistics for non-statisticians. *BMJ*. **315**: 422–5.

Greenhalgh T (1997) The Medline database. *BMJ*. **315** (19 July).

Griffiths R (1983) *NHS Management Inquiry*. DHSS, London.

Griffiths R (1983) *General Observations. Letter to Secretary of State on behalf of NHS Management Inquiry team*. 6 October.

Griffiths R (1991) Audit Commission Annual Lecture, 12 June 1991.

Griffiths R (1991) *Health Service Journal*. **20 June**.

Griffiths R (1992) Speech to British Association of Medical Managers, 3 June 1992.

Griffiths R (1992) Who cares? – management and the caring services. Abridged version of Jephcott Lecture (21 April 1992). *Journal of the Royal Society of Medicine*. **85**: 663–8.

Guba EG (1978) Toward a methodology of naturalistic inquiry in educational evaluation. Monograph 8. UCLA Center for the Study of Evaluation, Los Angeles.

Guba EG (1981) Criteria for assessing the trustworthiness of naturalistic inquiries. *Educational Communication and Technology Journal*. **29**: 75–92.

Gulleford J (1994) Preparing medical experts for the courtroom. No need to learn by trial and error. *BMJ*. **309**: 752–3.

Gunning R (1971) *The Technique of Clear Writing* (revised edition). McGraw Hill, New York.

Gusfield J (1960) Field work reciprocities in studying a social movement. In: R Adams and J Preiss (eds) *Human Organization Research*. Homewood, Dorsey.

Hadley R and Forster D (eds) (1993) *Doctors Managers – experiences in the front line of the NHS*. Longman Group, London.

Halpern ES (1983) Auditing naturalistic inquiries: the development and application of a model. Indiana University. Unpublished. In: Lincoln YS and Guba EG (1985) *Naturalistic Inquiry*. Sage Publications, California, p. 319.

Ham C (1999) The organisation of the NHS. In: *Wellard's NHS Handbook 1999/2000*. Section 1.2.

Ham C (1997) *Healthcare Reform*. Open University Press, Buckingham.

Hampden-Turner C (1990) *Charting the Corporate Mind: from dilemma to strategy*. Blackwell, Oxford.

Handy CB (1985) *Understanding Organizations* (3e). Penguin, London.

Handy CB (1991) *Gods of Management* (3e). Business Books, London.

Hanlon MD and Gladstein DL (1984) Improving the quality of work life in hospitals. *Hospital and Health Services Administration*. **September/October**: 94–107.

Harris D, Peyton R and Walker M (1996) Teaching in different situations. In: *Training the Trainers: learning and teaching*. Royal College of Surgeons, London.

Harris TA (1970) *I'm OK, You're OK*. Pan, London.

Harrison EF (1987) *The Managerial Decision Making Process*. Houghton-Mifflin, Boston.

Harrison S (1988) *Managing the National Health Service – shifting the frontier?* Chapman & Hall, London.

Harrison S (1996/97) NHS management. *NAHAT NHS handbook 1996/97*. Section 1.5

Harrison S, Hunter DJ and Pollitt C (1990) *The Dynamics of British Health Policy*. Unwin Hyman, London.

Harrison S and Pollitt C (1994) *Controlling Health Professionals*. Open University Press, Buckingham.

Hayek FA (1960) *The Constitution of Liberty*. Routledge & Kegan Paul, London.

HC(81)5 (part 3) *Complaints Relating to the Exercise of Clinical Judgement by Hospital Medical and Dental Staff*.

HC(88)37 *Hospital Complaints Procedure Act* 1985.

Heegaard M (1991) *When Someone Very Special Dies: children can learn to cope with grief*. Woodland, Minneapolis.

Heirs B and Farrell P (1989) *The Professional Decision Thinker. Our new management priority*. Grafton, London.

Heron J (1981) Philosophical basis for a new paradigm. In: P Reason and P Rowan (eds) *Human Inquiry*. Wiley, Chichester.

Heron J (1989) Validity in co-operative inquiry. In: R Reason (ed) *Human Inquiry in Action*. Sage, London.

Herzberg F (1966) *Work and the Nature of Man*. World Publishing Co, Evanston, Illinois.

Heys R (1991) Code of conduct needed to keep managers in line. *Hospital Doctor*. **5 December**: 28.

Heyssell RM, Gaintner JR, and Kues IW *et al.* (1984) Decentralised management in a teaching hospital. *The New England Journal of Medicine*. **310(22)**: 1477–1480.

Hickson DJ and Thomas MW (1969) Professionalisation in Britain, a preliminary measurement. *Sociology*. **3(1)**: 37–53.

Higgins J (1988) *The Business of Medicine*. Macmillan, Basingstoke.

Hirst DK and Clements RV (eds) (1995) *Clinical Directors Handbook*. Churchill Livingstone, London.

HMSO (1989) *Government White Paper. Working for Patients*. HMSO, London.

HMSO (1990) *Select Committee on the Parliamentary Commissioner for Administration. Third Report*. HMSO, London.

HMSO (1993) *The Children's Act Report 1993*. HMSO, London.

HMSO (1994) *What Seems to be the Matter?: communication between hospitals and patients*. HMSO, London.

HMSO (1994) *The Government's Expenditure Plans, 1994–5, 1996–7*. HMSO, London.

HMSO (1996) *The National Health Service: a service with ambition*. HMSO, London.

HMSO (1997) *The New NHS. Modern. Dependable*. HMSO, London.

Hocking J (1991) Managing in the Market Place: universities and institutional change in the late 1980s and early 1990s. University of Warwick. Unpublished.

Hoffenberg R (1987) *Clinical Freedom. Rock Carling Lecture*. Nuffield Provincial Hospitals Trust, London.

Hoffenberg R (1991) *The Harveian Oration*. Royal College of Physicians, London.

Holahan J, Moon M and Welch P *et al* (1991) An American approach to health system reform. *JAMA*. **265(19)**: 2537–40.

Honigsbaum F (1990) The evolution of the NHS. *BMJ*. **301**: 694–9.

Hood CA, Hope T and Dove P (1998) Videos, photographs, and patient consent. *BMJ*. **316**: 1009–11.

Hospital Service Manager (1997) Legal rulings on consent to treatment. Issue No. 21, 18 July.

HSG(95)13 *Revised and expanded Patient's Charter*.

Hughes V (1990) *English Language Skills*. Macmillan, London.

Human Resources Management (1996) *Manager Update*. **8(1)**: 23–5.

Hunt RG, Gurrslin O and Roach JL (1958) Social status and psychiatric service in a child guidance clinic. *American Sociological Review.* **23** (1 February): 81–3.

Hunter D (1992) From hierarchies to partnerships. *NHS Management Executive News.* **53**: 8.

Hunter DH and Fairfield G (1997) Managed care – disease management. *BMJ.* **315**: 50–3.

Hunter RB (1972) *Report of the Working Party on Medical Administrators.* DHSS. HMSO, London.

IHSM NHSTD (1994) *Managing for Quality. Management Education Scheme by Open Learning. Certificate Programme. Managing Health Services. Book 16.* Open University Press, Buckingham.

Illich I (1976) *Medical Nemisis: the expropriation of health.* Phantom Books, New York.

Inglehart JK (1983) The British National Health Service under the Conservatives. *New England Journal of Medicine.* **309**: 1264–8.

Inglehart JK (1984) The British National Health Service under the Conservatives – Part II. *New England Journal of Medicine.* **310**: 63–7.

IPM (1991) *The IPM Equal Opportunities Code.* Institute of Personnel Management, London.

Jacobs MO (1978) Administrators, boards, physicians must help change health system. *Hospitals.* **52(15)**: 78–80.

Jaques E (1976) *A General Theory of Bureaucracy.* Heinemann, London.

Jaques E (1978) *Health Services.* Heinemann, London.

Jaques E (1978) *Teams and Leadership. Health Services.* Heinemann, London.

Jarrold K (1992) From hierarchies to partnerships. *NHS Management Executive News.* **53**: 8.

Johnson TJ (1972) *Professions and Power.* Macmillan, London.

Jones H (1995) Textbook of management for doctors. In: T White (ed) *Engaging Doctors in Management.* Churchill Livingstone, London.

Jynton RP (1975) Boundaries in health care systems. *Journal of Applied Behavioural Science.* **11(2)**: 250.

Kaluzny AD and Hernandez SR (1988) Organizational change and innovation. In: SM Shortell and AD Kaluzney (eds) *Health Care Management: a text in organization theory and behaviour* (2e). Wiley, New York.

Kant I (1969) In: H Blumer (ed) *Symbolic Interactionism: perspective and method.* Prentice-Hall, New Jersey.

Kanter MR (1989) *When Giants Learn to Dance.* Unwin Hymans Ltd, London.

Kennedy I and Grubb A (1994) *Medical Law Text and Materials.* Butterworth, London.

Kieffer GD (1988) *The Strategy of Meetings.* Judy Piatkus, London.

King Edward's Hospital Fund (1985) *NHS Management Perspectives for Doctors*. King Edward's Hospital Fund, London.

King Edward's Hospital Fund (1990) *Equal Opportunities Task Force. Racial Equality: Hospital Doctors Selection Procedures*. King Edward's Hospital Fund, London.

King's Fund (1995) *Tackling Inequalities in Health – an agenda for action*. King's Fund, London.

Kirby J (1991) The hard up story of yesterday's trusts. *BMA News Review*. **3**: 19.

Klauser HA (1987) *Writing on Both Sides of the Brain*. Harper Collins, San Francisco.

Klein R (1985) Who makes the decisions in the NHS? In: *NHS Management Perspectives for Doctors*. King Edward's Hospital Fund, London.

Klein R (1989) *The Politics of The NHS* (2e). Longman, Harlow, Essex.

Klein R (1990) The state and the profession: the politics of the double bed. *BMJ*. **301**: 700.

Kliny R (1992) *Managing Clinical Services: decentralisation in action*. International Perspectives Conference, September 1992, London.

Knibbs J and Sellick R (1991) Tell them I'm in a meeting. *Health Service Journal*. **11 April**.

Kogan K *et al* (1978) *The Workings of the National Health Service. Research Paper No.1 Royal Commission on the NHS*. HMSO, London.

Kolb DA, Rubin IM and MacIntyre JM (1984) *Organizational Psychology – an experiential approach to organizational behaviour* (4e). Prentice-Hall, Englewood Cliffs, New Jersey.

Kotter JP (1977) Power dependence and effective management. *Harvard Business Review*. **July-August**: 125–36.

Kotter JP (1978) Power, success, and organizational effectiveness. Organizational dynamics. *American Management Association*. **Winter**: 27–40.

Kouzes JM and Mico PR (1979) Domain theory: an introduction to organizational behaviour in human service organizations. *Journal of Applied Behavioural Science*. **15(4)**: 449–68.

Ladd J (1957) *The Structure of a Moral Code*. Harvard University Press, Cambridge.

Lane J (1991) *Evaluation of Management Development for Hospital Consultants*. Jack Lane Associates, Ware.

Lane RE (1966) The decline of politics and ideology in a knowledgeable society. *American Sociological Review*. **31 October**.

Larkin G (1983) *Occupational Monopoly and Modern Medicine*. Tavistock, London.

Leathard A (1990) *Health Care Provision – past, present and future*. Chapman & Hall, London.

Lee-Potter J (1991) *BMA News Review*. **12 January**.

Leigh A (1991) *Effective Change*. Institute of Personnel Management, London.

Leitko TA and Szczerbacki D (1987) Why traditional OD strategies fail in professional bureaucracies. *Organizational Dynamics*. **15**: 52–65.

Levitt R and Wall A (1984) *The Reorganised Health Service* (3e). Chapman and Hall, London.

Light DW (1991) Observations on the NHS reforms: an American perspective. *BMJ*. **303**: 568–70.

Light DW (1997) The real ethics of rationing. *BMJ*. **315**: 112–15.

Lincoln & Louth NHS Trust (1996) *Breaking Bad News: guidelines for best practice*.

Lincoln YS and Guba EG (1985) *Naturalistic Inquiry*. Sage, California.

Lindenfield G (1993) *Managing Anger*. Thorsons, London.

Lindley RI (1998) Thrombolytic treatment for acute ischaemic stroke: consent can be ethical. *BMJ*. **316**: 1005–7.

Llewellyn K and Hoebel EA (1941) *The Cheyenne Way*. University of Oklahoma Press, Norman.

Lofland J (1976) *Doing Social Life*. Wiley, New York.

Longest BB (1990) *Management Practices for the Health Professional*. Appleton & Lange, Norwalk.

Loudon ISL (1979) *Trends in General Practice*. Royal College of General Practitioners, London.

Loveridge R and Starkey K (eds) (1992) *Continuity and Crisis in the NHS: the politics of design and innovation in health care*. Open University Press, Buckingham.

Lowry S (1992) Student selection. *BMJ*. **305**: 1352–4.

Lowry S (1993) *Medical Education*. BMJ Publishing Group, London.

Macauly TB (1991) *Meetings are central to your own career success and effective management*. In: K Blanchard and S Johnson (eds) *The One Minute Manager*. Collins, London.

McClure L (1985) Organization development in the healthcare setting. *Hospital and Health Services Administration*. **July/August**: 55–64.

McKeigue PM, Richards JDM and Richards P (1990) Effects of discrimination by sex and race on the early careers of British medical graduates during 1981–7. *BMJ*. **301**: 961–4.

McLean S (1997) EL(97)32 *Consent to Treatment – law and ethics in medicine*. Glasgow University, Glasgow.

Mangham IL (1978) *Interactions and interventions in organizations*. Wiley, Bath.

Mangham IL and Pye A (1991) *The Doing of Managing*. Blackwell, Oxford.

Mannheim K (1936) *Ideology and Utopia*. Harcourt, New York.

Maquire P (1990) Can communication skills be taught? *British Journal of Hospital Medicine.* **43**: 215–16.

Marshall J (1981) Making sense as a personal process. In: P Reason and J Rowan (eds) *Human Inquiry.* Wiley, Chichester.

Marteau TM *et al* (1990) Resuscitation: experience without feedback increases confidence but not skill. *BMJ.* **300**: 849–50.

Maruyama M (1978) In: P Reason and J Rowan (eds) *Human Inquiry* (1981). Wiley, Chichester.

Mascie-Taylor HM, Pedler MJ and Winkless AJ (1993) *Doctors & Dilemmas: a study of 'ideal types' of doctor/managers and an evaluation of how these could support values of clarification for doctors in the health service.* NHSTD, Bristol.

Maslow A (1972) Synergy in society and the individual. In: *The Farther Reaches of Human Nature.* The Viking Press, New York.

Massarik F (1981) The interviewing process re-examined. In: P Reason and J Rowan (eds) *Human Inquiry.* Wiley, Chichester.

Maxwell R (1992) Talk given at Managing Clinical Services: decentralisation in action conference. September 1992, London.

Maxwell R (1992) Speech at Workshop of Royal College Physicians. November 1992, London.

Maxwell R (1992). *Personal Communication.*

Maxwell R (1993) *The Role of Hospital Consultants in Clinical Directorates. The synchromesh report.* Royal College of Physicians, London.

Meadows R and Mitchels B (1989) Medical Reports. *BMJ.* **299**: 616–17.

Merrison AW (1975) Report of Committee of Inquiry into the Regulation of the Medical Profession. Secretary of State for Social Services. HMSO, London.

Migue J and Belanger G (1974) *The Price of Health.* Macmillan of Canada, Toronto.

Miles MB (1979) Qualitative data as an attractive nuisance: The problem of analysis. *Admin Sci Quarterly.* **24**: 590–610.

Millar B (1991) Clinicians as managers: medics make their minds up. *Health Service Journal.* **21 February**: 17.

Miller SM (1952) The participant-observer and 'over-rapport'. *American Sociological Review.* **17**: 97-9.

Mills I (1987) *Resource Management Feedback.* DHSS, London.

Mintzberg H (1973) *The Nature of Managerial Work.* Harper and Row, New York.

MoH (1948) *Report of the Interdepartmental Committee on the Remuneration of Consultants and Specialists.* HMSO, London.

MoH (1967) *First Report of the Joint Working Party on the Organisation of Medical Work in Hospitals.* HMSO, London.

Morgan G (1986) *Images of Organization.* Sage, London and California.

Mullins LJ (1998) *Management and Organisational Behaviour* (5e). Financial Times/Prentice Hall, London.

Musch K (1992) Talk given at Managing Clinical Services – decentralisation in action conference. September 1992, London.

Myrdal G (1944) *An American Dilemma. Appendix 2.* Harper, New York.

Nadler DA and Tichy NM (1982) The limitations of traditional intervention techniques in health care organizations. In: N Marguiles and JD Adams (eds) *Organizational Development in Health Care Organizations.* Addison-Wesley, Reading, MA.

Nelson MJ (1989) *Managing Health Professionals.* Chapman and Hall, London.

Neuberger J (1991) *Caring for Dying People of Different Faiths* (2e). Mosby, London.

NHS Management Executive (1990) *NHS Trusts: a working guide.* HMSO, London.

NHSE (1990) *A Guide to Consent for Examination.* NHSE, London.

NHSE (1994) *The Evolution of Clinical Audit.* NHSE, London.

NHSE (1994) *Developing NHS Purchasing and GP Fundholding: towards a primary care-led NHS.* NHS Executive, Leeds.

NHSE (1995) *Priorities and Planning Guidance for the NHS: 1999/2000.* NHSE, Leeds.

NHSE (1996) *A Guide to the National Health Service.* NHSE Communications Unit.

NHSE (1998) *A Guide to Specialist Registrar Training.* Department of Health, London.

NHSME (1991) *Framework of Audit for Nursing Services: guidance document*, EL(91)72. NHS Management Executive.

NHSME (1991) *NHS Management Executive, Equal Opportunities in Recruitment and Selection Procedures; Doctors and Dentists in the Hospital and Community Health Service.* HMSO, London.

NHSME (1994) *Report of the Joint Working Party on the Review of Appointment of Consultants, London*, EL(93)94. HMSO, London.

NHSTA (1989) *Doctors and Management Development: policy proposals from the National Health Service Training Authority.* NHSTA, Bristol.

Nichol D (1991) *BMA News Review.* **17(1)**: 10.

Nolan, Lord (1995) *First Report of the Committee on Standards in Public Life.* HMSO, London.

O'Brien E (1985) Prepare a curriculum vitae. In: *How to Do It.* Vol. 1 (2e). BMJ Publishing, London.

O'Connor M (1991) *Writing Successfully in Science.* Harper Collins, London.

O'Connor M (1995) *Editing Scientific Books and Journals*. Pitman Medical, London.

O'Donnell M (1997) Write for Money. In: *How to Do It*. Vol. 2. BMJ Publishing, London.

Øvretveit J (1995) *Purchasing for Health: health services management*. Open University Press, Buckingham.

Paice F, Collas D and Weightman J (1996) On-site modular training. *British Journal of Hospital Medicine*. **51(1,2)**.

Parker R (1993) *Healthcare Management*. **January**: 56–7.

Parston G (1986) *Managers as Strategists*. King Edward's Hospital Fund, London.

Pater JE (1981) *The Making of the National Health Service*. King's Fund, London.

Paton A (1985) Write a paper. In: *How to Do It*. Vol. 1 (2e). BMJ Publishing, London.

Paton C (1992) *Competition and Planning in the NHS – The danger of unplanned markets*. Chapman & Hall, London.

Peckham S and Winters M (1996) Unequal approach . . . community-based primary health care. *Nursing Times*. **March**: 20–6.

Peel M (1992) *Career Development and Planning*. McGraw-Hill International, UK.

Pellegrino ED (1972) The changing matrix of clinical decision-making in the hospital. In: BS Georgopoulis (ed) *Organization Research on Health Care Institutions*. Institute for Social Research, The University of Michigan, Michigan.

Pellegrino ED (1990) The relationship of autonomy and integrity in medical ethics. In: P Allebeck and B Jansson (eds) *Ethics in Medicine*. Raven Press, New York.

Pencheon D (1997) Will you blossom in public health medicine? *Consultant in Public Health Medicine BMJ Classified Section*. **21 June**.

Perros C (1978) *Complex Organizations*. Foresman, Glenview.

Perrow CB (1961) Organizational prestige: some functions and dysfunctions. *American Journal of Sociology*. **66(4)**: 335–41.

Perrow CB (1980) 'Zoo Story' or life in the organizational sandpit. In: G Salaman and K Thompson (eds) *Control and Ideology in Organizations*. Open University Press, Buckingham.

Perucci R (1973) Engineering: professional servant of power. In E Friedson (ed) *Professions and Their Prospects*. Sage, London.

Petchey R (1986) The Griffiths reorganisation of the NHS Fowerlism by stealth? *Critical Social Policy*. 87–101.

Peters T (1989) *Thriving on Chaos*. Pan Books, London.

Pettigrew A, Ferlie E and McKee L (1992) *Shaping Strategic Change, London. Making Change in Large Organizations. The Case of the NHS*. Sage, London.

Pfeiffer WJ (1982) Reprinted from: JW Pfeiffer and LD Goodstein (eds) *The 1982 Annual for Facilitators, Trainers, and Consultants.* University Associates, San Diego, CA.

Phillips DC (1985) After the wake: postpositivistic educational thought. *Educational Researcher.* **12**: 4–12.

Plovnick MS (1982) Structural interventions for health care systems' organizational development. Organizational development. In: N Margulies and JD Adams (eds) *Health Care Systems.* Addison-Wesley, Reading, MA.

Pollitt C, Harrison S and Hunter D *et al* (1988) The reluctant managers: clinicians and budgets in the NHS. *Financial Accountability & Management.* **4(3)**: 213–33.

Pope C (1991) Trouble in store: some thoughts on the management of waiting lists. *Sociology of Health and Illness.* **13**: 193–212.

Pope C and Mays N (1994) Opening the black box: an encounter in the corridors of health research. *BMJ.* **306**: 315–18.

Pouvourville G de (1989) Differences in the approaches of the doctor, manager, politician and social scientist in health care controversies – hospital case-mix management methods: an illustration of the manager's approach in health care controversies. *Soc Sci Med.* **29**: 341–9.

Power L (1998) Trial subjects must be fully involved in design and approval of trials. *BMJ.* **316**: 1003–4.

Pratt J (1995) *Practitioner and Practices: a conflict of values.* Radcliffe Medical Press, Oxford.

Prior J (1994) *Handbook of Training and Development* (2e). Gower/ITD, Aldershot.

Quick TL (1992) *Successful Team Building.* Amacom, New York.

Rapoport RN (1970) Three dilemmas of action research. *Human Relations.* **23(6)**: 499–513.

Rawlinson, Kelly and Whittlestone (1992) *The Shape of Things to Come.* A discussion paper on *The Hospital of the Future.* Commissioned by Regional Estates Managers Group, London.

RCN (1986) Interim guidance on implementing the new NHS complaints procedure. NHS Confederation briefing no. 91. Dealing with Complaints: Guidance for Good Practice. Issues in Nursing and Health Series, Royal College of Nursing.

RCS (1996) *Training the Trainers.* The Royal College of Surgeons of England. Raven Department of Education, London.

Reason P and Rowan J (1981) *Human Inquiry. Issues of validity in new paradigm research.* Wiley, Chichester.

Redfield R (1960) *The Little Community.* University of Chicago and Myrdal, Chicago.

Reeves D, Reid A and White A (1995) 'If it's Tuesday, this must be Shepton Mallet'. Taking ENT into the Community. *ENT News.* **4(2)**: 37.

Reich CA (1970) *The Greening of America. How the youth revolution is trying to make America liveable.* Random House, New York.

Reid A, Wall A and White A (1991) A wand for Cinderella: managing audiology services in a district health authority. *Health Services Journal*. **21 March**: 21.

Reid N (1993) *Healthcare Research by Degrees*. Blackwell Scientific Publications, London.

Reid T and David A (1995) Community nursing practice management and teamwork. *Nursing Times*. **December**.

Resource Management Feedback (1987) *The Resource Management Initiative*. **1** (August).

Riseborough PA and Walter M (1988) *Management in Health Care*. John Wright/Butterworth and Co., Bath.

Roberts REI (1994) The trials of an expert witness. *Journal of the Royal Society of Medicine*. **87**: 628–31.

Rosen G (1972) In: R Guest *The role of the doctor in institutional management*. In BS Georgopoulos (ed) *Organizational Research on Health Management*. Institute for Social Research, University of Michigan, Michigan.

Ross AP (1990) *Clinical Directors – a clinician's view. The Future of Acute Services. Doctors as Managers*. King's Fund Centre, London.

Rowbottom RW (1978) Professionals in Health and Social Services' Organizations. In: E Jacques (ed) *Health Services*. Heinemann, London.

Rowbottom RW *et al.* (1973) *Hospital Organization*. Heinemann, London.

Rubin I, Plovnick M and Fry R (1974) Initiating planned change in health care systems. *Journal of Applied Behavioural Science*. **10(1)**: 107–24.

Rubin I, Plovnick M and Fry R (1977) The role of the consultant in initiating planned change: A case study in health care systems. In: WW Burk (ed) *Current Issues and Strategies in Organization Development*. Human Sciences Press, New York.

Russell B (1958) *Portraits from Memory*. Allen & Unwin, London.

Sabin JE (1992) Mind the gap: reflections of an American health maintenance organisation doctor on the new NHS. *BMJ*. **305**: 514–16.

Sanford N (1981) A model for action research. In: P Reason and J Rowan (eds) *Human Inquiry*. Wiley, Chichester.

Sayles LR (1964) *Managerial Behaviour. Administration in complex organization*. McGraw-Hill, New York.

Schneller ES and Weiner TS (1985) The MD-JD revised. A sociological analysis of the cross-educated professionals in the decade of the 1980s. *Journal of Legal Medicine*. **6(3)**: 337–72.

Schon DA (1991) *The Reflective Practitioner: how professionals think in action*. The Academic Publishing Group, Aldershot.

Schulz R and Harrison S (1983) *Teams and Top Managers in the NHS, A Survey and Strategy. No 41*. King's Fund Centre Project Paper, London.

SCOPME (1990) *Medical Audit – educational implications*. SCOPME, London.

SCOPME (1996) *Appraising Doctors and Dentists in Training: a working paper for consultation*. SCOPME, London.

Scott WR (1965) Reactions to supervision in a heteronomous professional organization. *Administrative Science Quarterly*. **10**: 65–81.

Scriven M (1971) Objectivity and subjectivity in educational research. In LG Thomas (ed) *Philosophical Redirection of Educational Research* (71st Yearbook of the National Society for the Study of Education, part 1). University of Chicago Press, Chicago.

Scrivens E (1988) Doctors and managers: never the twain shall meet? *BMJ*. **296**: 1754–5.

Scwartz P and Ogilvy J (1980) *The Emergent Paradigm: changing patterns of thought and belief. Analytical Report No 7, Values and Lifestyles Program*. SRI International, California.

Shaw CD (1989) *Medical Audit. A hospital handbook*. King's Fund Centre, London.

Shaw CD (1989) *Guidelines for Medical Audit*. King's Fund Centre, London.

Shaw CD and Costain DW (1989) Guidelines for medical audit: seven principles. *BMJ*. **299**: 498–9.

Shields R and Leinster SJ (1993) *Position Paper on Clinical Directorates: a guide for surgeons*. Royal College of Surgeons of Edinburgh, Edinburgh.

Shortell SM, Morrison EM and Friedman B (1990) *Strategic Choices for America's Hospitals*. Jossey Bass, San Francisco.

Shortland M and Gregory J (1991) *Communicating Science*. Longman, Harlow.

Sieber JE (1992) *Planning Ethically Responsible Research*. Sage Publications, London.

Simendinger EA and Pasmore W (1984) Developing partnerships between physicians and healthcare executives. *Hospital and Health Services Administration*. **29**(Nov/Dec): 21–35.

Simmons J (1996) Management 2000 – the vision. John Simmons Lecture. *British Journal of Administrative Management*. **July/August**: 8–10.

Simpson J (1992) *Clinical Directorates Survey*. British Association of Medical Managers, Cheadle.

Simpson J and Scott T (1997) Beyond the call of duty. Report of a national survey carried out in 1996. *Health Service Journal*. **8 May**.

Sims DBP (1981) From ethogeny to endogeny: how participants in research projects can end up doing research on their own awareness. In: P Reason and J Rowan (eds) *Human Inquiry*. Wiley, Chichester.

Sims DBP (1987) From harmony to counterpoint. Organization analysis and development; a social construction of organizational behaviour. In: IL Mangham (ed) *Organization Analysis and Development*. Wiley, Chichester.

Singer EJ (1974) *Effective Management Coaching*. IPM, London.

Skynner ACR (1976) *One Flesh: separate persons. Principles of family and marital psychotherapy.* Constable, London.

Smith AJ and Preston D (1996) Communications between professional groups in an NHS trust hospital. *Journal of Management in Medicine.* **10(2)**: 31–9.

Smith GW (1984) *Towards an Organisation Theory for the NHS.* Health Services Manpower Review.

Smith HL (1958) Two lines of authority: the hospital's dilemma. In: EG Jaco (ed) *Patients, Physicians and Illness.* The Free Press, New York.

Smith MJ (1975) *When I Say No I Feel Guilty.* Bantam, London.

Snell J (1997) Feudal relationships – the chair and the chief executive. *Health Management.* **August**.

Speller SR (1971) *Law Relating to Hospitals and Kindred Institutions* (7e). Chapman & Hall, London.

Spurgeon P and Barwell F (1991) *Implementing Change in the NHS: a practical guide for managers.* Chapman & Hall, London.

Stansbie P (1996/97) *Health Authorities and NHS Purchasing. NAHAT NHS handbook 1996/97.* Section 2.4. The purchaser/provider relationship.

Stewart R (1967) *Managers and their Jobs.* Macmillan, London. Also In: *Contracts in Management.* McGraw-Hill, London.

Stewart R (1982) *Choices for the Manager.* McGraw-Hill, Maidenhead.

Stewart R (1986) *Involving Doctors in GM.* Templeton Series. Paper No 5. NHSTA, Bristol.

Stewart R (1989) *Leading in the NHS. A practical guide.* Macmillan Press, Basingstoke.

Stewart R and Dobson S (1988) Griffiths in theory and practice: a research assessment. *Journal of Health Administration Education.* **6(3)**: 503–14.

Strong P and Robinson J (1990) *The NHS – under new management.* Open University Press, Buckingham.

Strunk W and White EB (1979) *The Elements of Style* (3e). Macmillan, New York.

Sumners JW (1981) Money health and the health care industry. *Hospital and Health Services Administration.* **Winter**: 7–24.

Susman GI and Evered RD (1978) An assessment of the scientific merits of action research. *Admin Sci Quarterly.* **23**: 582–603.

Sutton M (1997) How to get the best health outcome for a given amount of money. *BMJ.* **315** (5 July).

Templeton Series on DGM's Issue Study 5 (1986) *Managing with Doctors. Working together?* NHS Training Authority. The Academic Publishing Group, Aldershot.

Thome C (1991) Chartered Institute of Public Finance and Accountancy Conference in June 1991. Reported in *Health Service Journal*. **20 June**.

Thompson A (1995) The case for caution in a courtroom fight. *Hospital Doctor*. **January**: 24.

Thompson D (1987) Coalitions and conflict in the NHS, some implications for management. *Sociology of Health and Illness*. **9(2)**: 125–53.

Thompson JD (1972) *Organizations in Action*. McGraw-Hill, New York.

Thompson R (1996) Quality in health care. In: A White (ed) *Textbook of Management for Doctors*. Churchill Livingstone, Edinburgh.

Timbs O and White T (1993) Clinician's questionnaire. *Healthcare Management*. **1(3)**: 33–6.

Timbs O and White T (1993) Yes, you are managing. *Health Care Management*. **1(5)**: 16–18.

Tobias JS (1998) Changing the BMJ's position on informed consent would be counter-productive. *BMJ*. **316**: 1001–2.

Toghill PJ (1992) Merit awards. *Hospital Update Plus*. **October**: 140–2.

Tolliday H (1978) Clinical autonomy. In: E Jaques (ed) *Health Services*. Heinemann, London.

Tomlinson B (1992) *Report of the Inquiry into London's Health Services, Medical Education and Research*. HMSO, London.

Townley B (1991) Selection and appraisal: reconstituting 'social relations'. In: J Storey *New Perspectives on Human Resource Management*. Routledge, London.

Toynbee P (1977) *Hospital*. Hutchinson, London.

Trapp R (1997) *Time to nurture those soft skills*. Roger Daniel Coleman, Independent tabloid, London.

Turrill T, Wilson D and Young K (1991) *The Characteristics of Excellent Doctors in Management* NHS Management Executive, Resource Management Unit. Turrill, Thirsk.

Turrill T, Wilson D and Young K (1993) *Transforming Doctors' Dilemmas*. Turrill, Thirsk.

Vidich A and Bensman J (1960) The validity of field data. In: R Adams and J Preiss (eds) *Human Organization Research*. Dorsey, Homewood.

Vinter RD (1959) The structure of service. In: AJ Kahn (ed) *Issues in American Social Work*. Columbia University Press, New York.

Vinter RD (1963) Analysis of treatment organizations. *Social Work*. **July**: 3–15.

Wall A (1999) NHS boards and their functions. In: *Wellard's NHS Handbook 1999/2000*.

Ward S (1995) Laying down the law on medical evidence. *BMA News Review*. **June**: 21–2.

Warden J (1991) The manager is king. *BMJ*. **302**: 1298.

Warnock M (1998) Informed consent – a publisher's duty. *BMJ*. **316**: 1002–3.

Wax R (1960) Reciprocity in field work. In: R Adams and J Preiss (eds) *Human Organization Research*. Dorsey, Homewood.

Weber M (1947) *The Theory of Social and Economic Organization*. Oxford University Press, Oxford.

Weed LL (1997) New connections between medical knowledge and patient care. *BMJ*. **315**: 231–5.

Weisbord MR (1976) Why organization development hasn't worked (so far) in medical centers. *Health Care Management Review*. **Spring**: 17–28.

Weisbord MR and Stoelwinder JU (1979) Linking physicians, hospital management, cost containment and better patient care. *Health Care Management Review*. **4(2)**.

Welborne IWB (1990) The Management of change. *British Journal of Hospital Medicine*. **44** (July): 53–5.

West PA (1988) *Understanding the NHS: a question of incentives*. King Edward's Hospital Fund, London.

Whale J (1984) *Put It In Writing*. JM Dent and Sons, London.

Wheeler SJ (1989) Health visitors' and social workers' perceptions of child abuse (dissertation). Unpublished. Bournemouth University.

White A (1990) My brilliant idea and what happened to it. *BMA News Review*. **16(11)**.

White A (1991) Be a journalist for a day . . . or more. *BMA News Review*. **17(8)**.

White A (1991) Managing with next to nothing. On being a clinical director. *BMA News Review*. **17(4)**.

White A (1992) *Making Medical Audit Effective. Module 7. Achieving Change through Audit*. Joint Centre for Medical Education, London.

White A (1992) *Management for Clinicians*. Edward Arnold, London.

White A (1993) Yes, you are managing. *Healthcare Management*. **May**.

White A (1993) The role of hospital consultants in management, decision making and change (dissertation). Unpublished. Bath University.

White A (1993). Managing the chair. In: *Management for Clinicians*. Edward Arnold, London.

White A (1993) Clinicians' questionnaire. *Healthcare Management*. **March**.

White A and Reid A (1995) If it's Tuesday, this must be Shepton Mallet. Taking ENT into the Community. *ENT News*. **4(2)**.

White A (1996) *Managing Meetings*. Churchill Livingstone, London.

White A (1996) *Textbook of Management for Doctors*. Churchill Livingstone, London.

White A and Gatrell J (1997) Management development for doctors' research in South and West Region. In: *Progress in Medical Management*. Churchill Livingstone, London.

White A and Gatrell J (1997) *Professional or Manager? Medical doctors in management in the UK National Health Service*. European Forum for Management Development.

Wilensky HL (1964) The professionalisation of everyone? *American Journal of Sociology*. **70**: 137–58.

Wiles R and Robinson J (1994) Teamwork in primary care: the views and experiences of nurses, midwives and health visitors. *Journal of Advanced Nursing*. **20(2)**.

Williams A (1985) *Medical Ethics: health service efficiency and clinical freedom*. Nuffield/York Portfolio No.2 Nuffield Provincial Hospitals Trust, London.

Wilson N (1946) *Municipal Health Services*. Allen and Unwin, London.

Wilson RN (1959/60) The physician's changing hospital role. *Human Organization*. **18**: 177–83.

Wilson (1994) *Being Heard, The Report of a Review Committee on NHS Complaints Procedures*. Wilson Committee, NHSEP

Winder E (1994) Prevention and control of clinical negligence. *Clinician in Management*. **3** suppl 1(5): 15.

Winkenwerder W and Ball JR (1988) Transformation of American health care. The role of the medical profession. *New England Journal of Medicine*. **318**: 317–19.

Wraith M and Casey A (1992) *New Management in Evolution*. Wraith Casey, Droitwich.

Wraith M and Casey A (1992) *Implementing Clinically Based Management. Getting Organisational Change Underway*. Wraith Casey, Droitwich.

Wright B (1991) *Sudden Death*. Churchill Livingstone, Edinburgh.

Wright B (1993) *Caring in Crisis* (2e). Churchill Livingstone, Edinburgh.

Wright B (1998) *Matter of Death and Life*. King Edward's Hospital Fund, London.

Zander AF, Cohen AR and Stotland E (1957) *Role Relations in Mental Health Professions*. University of Michigan Press, Michigan.

Index